100 Questions & Answers About Advanced and Metastatic Breast Cancer
Second Edition

Lillie D. Shockney, RN, BS, MAS

Administrative Director
Johns Hopkins Avon Foundation Breast Center
University Distinguished Service
Associate Professor of Breast Cancer
Johns Hopkins University School of Medicine
Departments of Surgery, Gynecology, and Obstetrics
Associate Professor
Johns Hopkins University School of Nursing
Baltimore, MD

Gary R. Shapiro, MD

Associate Professor
Department of Oncology
Johns Hopkins Sidney Kimmel Comprehensive Cancer Center
Johns Hopkins Avon Foundation Breast Center
Baltimore, MD

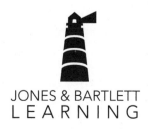

JONES & BARTLETT
L E A R N I N G

World Headquarters
Jones & Bartlett Learning
40 Tall Pine Drive
Sudbury, MA 01776
978-443-5000
info@jblearning.com
www.jblearning.com

Jones & Bartlett Learning books and products are available through most bookstores and online booksellers. To contact Jones & Bartlett Learning directly, call 800-832-0034, fax 978-443-8000, or visit our website, www.jblearning.com.

Substantial discounts on bulk quantities of Jones & Bartlett Learning publications are available to corporations, professional associations, and other qualified organizations. For details and specific discount information, contact the special sales department at Jones & Bartlett Learning via the above contact information or send an email to specialsales@jblearning.com.

The authors, editor, and publisher have made every effort to provide accurate information. However, they are not responsible for errors, omissions, or for any outcomes related to the use of the contents of this book and take no responsibility for the use of the products and procedures described. Treatments and side effects described in this book may not be applicable to all people; likewise, some people may require a dose or experience a side effect that is not described herein. Drugs and medical devices are discussed that may have limited availability controlled by the Food and Drug Administration (FDA) for use only in a research study or clinical trial. Research, clinical practice, and government regulations often change the accepted standard in this field. When consideration is being given to use of any drug in the clinical setting, the healthcare provider or reader is responsible for determining FDA status of the drug, reading the package insert, and reviewing prescribing information for the most up-to-date recommendations on dose, precautions, and contraindications, and determining the appropriate usage for the product. This is especially important in the case of drugs that are new or seldom used.

Production Credits

Executive Publisher: Christopher Davis
Managing Editor, Custom Projects: Kathy Richardson
Associate Production Editor: Jill Morton
Associate Marketing Manager: Katie Hennessy
Manufacturing and Inventory Control Supervisor:
  Amy Bacus
Composition: Spoke & Wheel

Cover Design: Carolyn Downer
Cover Images: Upper left, © Otnaydur/Dreamstime.com;
Upper right, © David Smith/Dreamstime.com;
Lower left, © Yuri/Dreamstime.com;
Lower right, © Feverpitched/Dreamstime.com
Printing and Binding: Malloy Incorporated
Cover Printing: Malloy Incorporated

Library of Congress Cataloging-in-Publication Data
Shockney, Lillie, 1953–
    100 questions & answers about advanced and metastatic breast cancer / by Lillie D. Shockney and Gary R. Shapiro. —2nd ed.
        p. cm.
    Includes bibliographical references and index.
    ISBN: 978-1-4496-4335-5
    1. Breast—Cancer—Popular works. 2. Metastasis—Popular works. I. Shapiro, Gary R. II. Title. III. Title: One hundred questions and answers about advanced and metastatic breast cancer.
    RC280.B8S494 2012
    616.99'449—dc22
                                                                        2011003458
6048

Printed in the United States of America
16 15 14   10 9 8 7 6 5 4 3

CONTENTS

Breast cancer remains the most feared disease among women. Receiving a diagnosis of stage IV breast cancer is a shock, and it affects you and everyone who loves you.

This book is designed to help you, and those who care about you, understand what metastatic breast cancer is and what treatment options there are. It will also help you make decisions regarding those treatment choices and help you plan for your future.

There are no magic bullets regarding treatment for this stage of disease. There is hope and with more research being completed every year, that hope grows.

This book contains the top 100 questions women ask to help them understand their disease, how best to cope with its treatment, and other matters that impact their life as they progress along with treatment. It is our hope that this information will be helpful for you and your loved ones.

Eleanor Roosevelt wrote years ago, "Yesterday is history; tomorrow is a mystery; today is a gift—that's why it's called 'the present.'" I believe Roosevelt's quote is an accurate summation of what women are experiencing on their journey with this disease.

Lillie Shockney, RN, BS, MAS
University Distinguished Service Associate Professor of Breast Cancer
18-year breast cancer survivor

PART ONE

Suspicions of Metastatic Breast Cancer

Does the diagnosis of metastatic breast cancer mean an instant death sentence?

How will my oncologist decide to treat my metastatic breast cancer?

I want to get under way with treatment immediately and everything is taking too long. Why can't I start treatment immediately?

More . . .

Chemotherapy

Treatment with drugs that kill cancer cells or make them less active. It is a form of systemic treatment.

Hormonal therapy

Treatment that blocks the effects of hormones upon cancers.

Targeted therapy

Cancer treatments that target specific characteristics of cancer cells, such as a protein, an enzyme, or the formation of new blood vessels. Targeted therapies don't harm normal, healthy cells.

Metastatic breast cancer

Cancer that has spread from the breast to other organ sites such as the liver, lung, bone, or brain.

Locally advanced disease

Stage III breast cancer.

Oncologist

A cancer specialist who helps determine treatment choices.

Remission

A decrease in or disappearance of signs and symptoms of cancer.

There is a very good possibility that you have already been told that you have breast **cancer** and have undergone treatment for it. You may have had surgery, **chemotherapy**, radiation, and maybe **hormonal therapy** or **targeted biologic therapy** and now you are being told that there is a chance that your new symptoms are related to **metastatic breast cancer**. You are not alone in feeling frightened and scared about hearing this news. Recurrence of breast cancer is the biggest fear for all breast cancer survivors. Though the risk of distant recurrence is highest during the first 2 years after treatment and affects more women with **locally advanced disease (stage III)** than with stage I or stage II disease, metastatic breast cancer can occur at any point in time after the original diagnosis. The only group that it is considered to not be at risk for metastatic breast cancer is women who had stage 0 or noninvasive breast cancer.

Once you've been diagnosed with metastatic breast cancer, risk level statistics don't have the same meaning. Having a small risk of developing metastatic disease doesn't change the current situation. If you've been diagnosed with or told that you might have metastatic breast cancer, it's serious for you. Every imaginable fear may be rushing through your mind. You may have come to the **oncologist's** office with complaints of back pain that you've been experiencing for the last 3 weeks that won't subside with over-the-counter pain relievers. Maybe you have headaches or some new symptom related to your breathing. Your symptoms may have triggered the doctor to order additional tests to determine if these symptoms are related to your original breast cancer diagnosis. Remember, many people can live for years with metastatic breast cancer. The cancer can be "active" sometimes, then go into **remission**. Let's walk through information about metastatic breast cancer together so that you are well informed and can participate in the decision-making about your treatment and care.

1. So what is metastatic breast cancer?

Breast cancer is referred to as **recurrent breast cancer** if it reappears after it was originally diagnosed and treated. Recurrence happens in two forms. There is **local recurrence**, which means that it came back in the breast where it originally started. There is also **distant recurrence** or metastatic breast cancer. In metastatic breast cancer, the cancer has returned to another part of the body, including distant organs such as the lungs, liver, bones, or brain. It is also known as stage IV breast cancer. The goal for treatment is control of the disease. Think of it as a chronic illness, like diabetes. If diabetics didn't watch their diet and take their insulin several times a day, they would not survive. This chronic illness works in a similar way. You take treatments regularly to keep the disease in control and, whenever possible, put it into remission so that it is not actively growing. At a minimum, the goal is to maintain good quality of life for the patient while also treating the disease so that it remains stable over time and doesn't progress. The goal is not cure, the goal is control. When breast cancer attacks other organs in the body, these organs can have difficulty doing their daily job—creating new blood **cells**, providing oxygen, metabolizing medicines, keeping our heart and lungs functioning properly, and other important processes required to sustain life.

There are some situations in which a patient is diagnosed with metastatic breast cancer at the time of their initial diagnosis. This is less common however. Most occur in the form of a distant recurrence some time after the patient's initial diagnosis and treatment.

Recurrent cancer

The disease has come back in spite of the initial treatment.

Local recurrence

The breast cancer has returned inside the breast after treatment was completed.

Distant recurrence

The breast cancer has been found now in another organ, such as the lungs, liver, bones, or brain. It is located outside of the breast and lymph nodes near the breast.

Cells

Basic elements of tissues; the appearance and composition of individual cells are unique to the tissue they compose.

Cancer is a disease of aging, and the incidence of breast cancer is increasing faster in older women than in younger women.

Incidence

The number of times a disease occurs within a population of people.

Tumor

A mass or lump of extra tissue.

Hormone receptor

A protein on the surface or inside a cell that connects to a certain hormone (estrogen or progesterone) and causes changes in the cell.

HER2 overexpression

An excess of a certain protein (HER2) on the surface of a cell that may be related to a high number of abnormal or defective cells.

Metastases, metastasize

The spread of cancer from one part of the body to another.

2. Does the diagnosis of metastatic breast cancer mean an instant death sentence?

No, it does not. However, it is true that a large number of women with stage IV breast cancer (metastatic breast cancer) will succumb to this disease. Still there are women who continue to live long and productive lives living in harmony with their disease—like someone who needs to keep their sugar levels in constant check.

Katie's comments:

I was in shock when I first heard that my cancer had returned and was in my bones. I had had a few aches and pains that lingered longer than usual but I never expected to hear this kind of news. Fortunately, this doesn't mean a death sentence like I assumed it would. Hormonal therapy may get this back into control the doctor said. My mission is to live a long life still with my family and I will continue to set goals for the future.

3. I have heard that breast cancer grows more slowly in older women and doesn't need to be treated. Is that true?

Cancer is a disease of aging, and the **incidence** of breast cancer is increasing faster in older women than in younger women. Older adults with cancer often have other chronic health problems and may be taking multiple medications, both of which can affect their cancer treatment plan. Misconceptions and prejudice often prevent older patients from getting the cancer treatment that they need.

The biology of breast cancer is different in older women than younger women. As patients age, their breast **tumors** more frequently express **hormone receptors** (estrogen, progesterone), they have lower rates of tumor cell growth, and lower **overexpression of HER2** (human epidermal growth factor receptor 2). Though these are usually thought of as favorable factors, most recent studies show no major age-related differences in breast cancer survival. In fact, older women with **metastases** often have more aggressive disease than their younger counterparts. Chronological age alone should not be the only factor used to determine how and when to use life-prolonging or **palliative** anti-cancer treatment. Despite advanced age, men and women who are relatively well often have a life expectancy that may exceed their life expectancy with breast cancer. The average 70-year-old woman is likely to live another 16 years. A similar 85-year-old can expect to live an additional 6 years and remain functionally independent for most of that time. Even an unwell 75-year-old probably will live five more years; long enough to experience symptoms and early death from metastatic breast cancer.

Since most older women have **estrogen or progesterone-receptor positive breast cancer**, hormonal therapy is often an excellent treatment option. **Aromatase inhibitors** (like anastrozole) work better and generally have fewer side effects than tamoxifen in postmenopausal women. On the other hand, they are associated with an increased risk of osteoporosis and related fractures. It is, therefore, important for oncologists to monitor the bone health of these women with **bone density (DEXA) scans**. The appropriate use of calcium and bisphosphonates is an important **adjunct** to the use of these agents. Elderly breast cancer patients are particularly susceptible to chemotherapy-induced **anemia, neutropenia,** mucositis, diarrhea, and dehydration. Though the side effects of cancer treatment are never less burdensome in the elderly, they can be managed by oncologists; especially geriatric oncologists, who work in teams with

Palliative care

Care to relieve the symptoms of cancer and to keep the best quality of life for as long as possible.

Estrogen/ progesterone-receptor positive cancer

Cancer that uses female hormones as a fuel to grow.

Aromatase inhibitor

Drugs that lower the amount of estrogen made in the body after menopause. This can slow or stop the growth of cancer that needs estrogen to grow.

Bone density (DEXA) scan

A test for osteoporosis and osteopenia.

Adjunct

A treatment that compliments another treatment.

Anemia

A condition in which the number of red blood cells is too low.

Neutropenia

An abnormally low number of a particular type of white blood cell called neutrophils.

others who specialize in the care of the elderly. With appropriate care, healthy older women do just as well with chemotherapy as younger women.

4. How will my oncologist decide how to treat my metastatic breast cancer?

Treatment of metastatic breast cancer can prolong life and enhance its quality, but there is no cure. Therefore, your oncologist's strategy is to get as much mileage out of each treatment regimen as possible. Since treatments with the fewest side effects are preferred, your oncologist will try to use hormonal therapies instead of chemotherapy, whenever reasonable. Of course, hormonal therapy is only an option if your breast cancer is estrogen or progesterone receptor positive.

Many women with hormone receptor positive breast cancer benefit from sequential hormone therapies when their disease progresses. Premenopausal women who have had anti-estrogen **adjuvant therapy** (usually tamoxifen) will typically be treated with an aromatase inhibitor (like anastrozole) after they are put into a postmenopausal state by an oophorectomy (surgically, or induced with **radiation therapy** or with medicines such as goserelin or leuprolide). Tamoxifen is an option for **first-line hormonal therapy** if you are premenopausal and have never received anti-estrogens, or it has been more than 1 year since you stopped taking them. An aromatase inhibitor (anastrozole, letrozole, exemestane) is the first-line hormonal therapy if you are postmenopausal. The anti-estrogen fulvestrant (Faslodex®) is available for the treatment of postmenopausal women with hormone receptor-positive metastatic breast cancer that has been previously treated with an anti-estrogen. Other hormone therapies include progestin (megestrol acetate),

Adjuvant therapy

Treatment given after the primary treatment to increase the chances of a cure.

Radiation therapy

The use of high-energy X-rays to kill cancer cells and shrink tumors.

First-line therapy

The first drug or set of drugs that you receive as your treatment.

androgens (fluoxymesterone), and high-dose estrogens (ethinyl estradiol).

Hormone therapy is especially useful in patients whose metastatic disease involves only bone or soft tissue. Though it is also useful in treating metastases to the vital organs (especially if there are no symptoms), chemotherapy will be recommended in these situations. Even if your metastases remain limited to the bone or soft tissue, once your cancer stops responding to hormonal therapy, your oncologist will have no other choice but to switch to chemotherapy. Of course, if your cancer is not estrogen receptor positive or progesterone receptor positive, chemotherapy is your only option.

If your breast cancer has a HER2 overexpression of the oncogene, your oncologist will probably recommend targeted therapy with trastuzumab (Herceptin), or, if you have already received trastuzumab (Herceptin), then using another agent, lapatinib (Tykerb). He can give trastuzumab to you as a single agent, but often will combine it with traditional **cytotoxic** chemotherapeutic agents like paclitaxel (Taxol). Trastuzumab can have debilitating heart toxicity, and your oncologist will need to make sure that you are not at risk before he administers this drug to you. Even if your tumor is HER2 positive, if you meet the criteria for hormonal therapy, most oncologists prefer to go that route before resorting to trastuzumab.

Cytotoxic
A term used to describe anything that kills cells.

Metastatic breast cancer is sensitive to many cytotoxic chemotherapy agents. The following are among those most commonly used as first-, second-, or subsequent line treatment. You could get these as single agents or in various combinations: paclitaxel, docetaxel, capecitabine, gemcitabine, vinorelbine, doxorubicin, epirubicin, pegylated liposomal doxorubicin, cyclophosphamide, fluorouracil, cisplatin, carboplatin, and eribulin mesylate.

Patients often ask what is the "best" treatment regimen. Oncologists will differ on how they answer that question. What they will all tell you is that there really is no good way of knowing without first trying. The order in which they choose to use these palliative agents will depend upon your overall health, the location of your metastases, and your track record with previous treatment regimens. Though results of clinical trials initially influences drug choice, after a certain point, the choice is more "art" and personal preference than "science."

The order in which they choose to use these palliative agents will depend upon your overall health, the distribution of your metastases, and your track record with previous treatment regimens.

5. My doctor waited for me to have symptoms before doing any scans. Couldn't he have found my cancer earlier if he did regular scans after my first diagnosis?

Scans

A technique to create images of specific parts of the body on a computer screen or on film.

There are tests, such as **scans**, that might detect the presence of cancer in other organs before symptoms appear. Research studies have confirmed that doing these tests does not improve the response to treatments used and thereby doesn't translate into prolonging someone's life. While that probably sounds strange, studies have shown it to be true. An additional issue is that performing routine scans and blood work can result in finding things that frighten the patient, only to learn after careful investigation the findings are normal and not cancer related. Scans cannot see microscopic disease that is starting to establish itself in another organ, either. Even a scan that shows no evidence of disease isn't really a guarantee that there aren't microscopic cells growing elsewhere that can't be detected at that time.

Your doctor will focus on the areas where you have symptoms. Shortness of breath would trigger a lung scan and chest X-ray; back pain would result in a **bone scan**, for example. A blood test called CA27/29 will likely be done, as well as some routine blood chemistries to provide additional information to assist the doctors in determining the underlying cause of your symptoms. It is becoming increasingly common to **biopsy** the organ site where the scans are showing the potential presence of breast cancer. Your doctor might order a bone, liver, lung, or brain biopsy. Having a **pathologist** have access to actual tissue from the organ provides a definitive diagnosis while enabling the oncology team to learn more about the cancer that has spread. When you were initially diagnosed, the cancer cells in your breast were tested for specific prognostic factors. These included hormone receptors, HER2 receptors, grade of the cells, size of the tumor, **Ki67** to measure its proliferation rate of the cells, and other measurements. The tissue biopsied from the organ site also is tested in a similar way. We used to assume that the cells that traveled from the breast to distant sites would have the exact same prognostic factors as they originally had. We now are learning from laboratory research that this may not be the case. When the cancer has traveled and spread, it might have converted from being hormone receptor positive to hormone receptor negative, for example. This information is critical to planning the right treatment options. The medicines and therapies prescribed are customized to work best on your specific cancer cells that have traveled out of the breast and gone to live elsewhere in your body.

Bone scan

An X-ray that looks for signs of metastasis to the bones.

Biopsy

A procedure in which cells are collected for microscopic examination.

Pathologist

A specialist trained to distinguish normal from abnormal cells.

Ki67

A molecule that can be easily detected in growing cells in order to gain an understanding of the rate at which the cells within a tumor are growing.

6. How long is it going to take before I know if I have metastatic breast cancer?

It may be challenging and frustrating for both you and your doctors that it can take a few days or even a couple of weeks to determine if you do, in fact, have metastatic breast cancer. As anxiety provoking as that may seem, it's important that tests are done accurately, correlated with other findings, and in some cases, biopsies done to confirm the diagnosis, before any treatment can be planned. This time frame, though long for you, is important so that the right things are done in the right way. Waiting a few more weeks will not alter how well you are going to do. The mission is control of the disease once it's confirmed. Knowing the pathology information and findings from scans and other X-rays is important in selecting the optimal treatment plan for you.

7. How did this happen? Should I have had more treatment originally when I was diagnosed?

This is a common question. Some women feel guilty; others angry. All are certainly in shock. If you decided against a treatment you were advised to have, don't second guess yourself. Hindsight is always 20/20. Stay focused and move forward. The question to ask yourself is "What do I need to do now to get control over this disease and live in harmony with it?" If you are feeling angry, that is okay. You may feel that have paid your dues to this disease and just found out you need to do it again, only perhaps in a scarier way. It's okay to grieve about it, be mad about it, as long as you keep moving forward with your doctors and nurses and plan your treatment.

8. I want to get under way with treatment immediately and everything is taking too long. Why can't I start treatment immediately?

It is in your best interest that all the test results and clinical findings are clearly understood and known before beginning treatment. There may be several different treatment options too for you to consider. You shouldn't feel rushed in making these very important decisions. Have thoughtful discussions with your oncology team. Each new doctor you see and talk to may give you new information. Remember, when you are scared and anxious you may not process information very clearly. It can be difficult to be patient, but planning the treatment that is in your best interest is a goal shared by your oncology team. Taking a few weeks to iron out the best strategy will help ensure that the most appropriate decisions have been made to give you the best opportunity for living in harmony with this disease. This is the time for thoughtful and wise decisions.

PART TWO

Ensuring You Are in Good Hands— Selecting the Oncology Team to Take Care of You

How do I know I'm receiving the best and most appropriate care for my current situation?

How can I participate in the decision-making about my treatment?

How do I select a medical oncologist who will be primarily responsible for my care and treatments?

More . . .

9. How do I know I'm receiving the best and most appropriate care for my current situation?

It would seem to make perfect sense to be taken care of by the oncology team who originally treated you for breast cancer. Your clinical situation is now much more serious than perhaps it was at that time. There are some steps you may want to take to ensure that this is the most appropriate team to continue managing your care.

You can't judge a breast center's quality based on the facility's advertisements.

You can't judge a breast center's quality based on the facility's advertisements. Sometimes it requires a lot of effort on your part (or someone else's, on your behalf) to do the necessary due diligence to ensure that you are in good hands. There are efforts under way by organizations like the National Consortium of Breast Centers to more clearly define what a "breast center" is and how to measure quality of care for patients undergoing diagnosis and treatment of breast cancer. Presently there are no standards that define what is meant by these terms. A breast center that is part of a National Cancer Institute (NCI)-designated cancer center is usually a wise choice. There are many services and programs that a patient should be seeking from a breast center when she is initially diagnosed and treated. For women dealing with metastatic breast cancer, there are some specific features that you want to be sure are available to you. They include:

1. *Patient empowerment.* It's important that you be given the knowledge you need to enable you to actively participate in the decisions about your care and treatment. Some physicians are reluctant to empower women in this way. Make sure this is understood as an expectation you have.

2. *Patient and family education.* Not only do you need to be educated, so does your family. You need to know what to expect, when, how, and why. You need easy access to someone who will be able to support you and respond to your questions as you take this critical journey. It is important to receive written literature as well as verbal information.

3. *Multidisciplinary case conferences.* The key advantage to having a multidisciplinary team approach is the special expertise each healthcare professional offers to the patient's unique situation. Centers that hold weekly breast cancer conferences can provide that. There may be times that your next steps for treatment decision-making are unclear to both you and your doctor. Your doctor can present your case to the entire team in this setting and get input on your behalf.

4. *Access to **clinical trials**.* This may be one of the most important times that you want to ensure you have access to clinical trials that may offer additional benefits to controlling this disease. These clinical trials would include all **phases** of research study.

5. *Medical oncologists.* You want to ensure that the medical oncologist taking care of you specializes in breast cancer and has expertise in women with metastatic disease.

6. *Radiation oncologists.* There may be a need for radiation during your treatment so you want to ensure that the radiation oncologist specializes in breast cancer and has expertise in treating women with metastatic disease.

7. *Pathologists.* Though you have been diagnosed and have your prognostic factors about the tumor, there may be times in which additional biopsies are needed.

Clinical trials

Research studies in which patients are offered the opportunity to try new innovative therapies (under careful observation) in order to help doctors identify the best treatments with the fewest side effects. These studies help improve the overall standard of care.

Phases

A series of steps followed in clinical trials.

For example, you may need biopsies of other organ sites. You want a facility that has pathologists who specialize in breast pathology because their accuracy is critical to planning your treatment.

8. *Pathology services.* Patients don't always think about this particular service but it is a very important one. The pathologist who looks at your tissue specimen determines the prognostic factors, and the rest of the team uses that information to formulate a treatment plan. Accuracy and completeness are critical. Some say that the pathologist "holds all the cards" because her opinion about what is on your pathology slides is critical information. We don't want to overtreat or undertreat a patient, but this happens every day because there are no clear standards regarding pathology interpretation. A breast center that has pathologists who specialize in breast pathology has an edge since they are likely to see higher volume than other pathologists. They have also made a commitment to specialize in breast disease. The pathology from other organ sites where the breast cancer may have spread will be compared to the original pathology found in the breast tumor itself. Sometimes it is discovered that the prognostic factors (like hormone receptors and HER2) have changed. This type of accuracy and preciseness is very important in planning the optimal treatment for your specific pathology situation.

9. *Urgent care needs.* When an urgent problem arises, such as spiking a fever, you need to have ready access to a healthcare professional who is easy to reach and who knows how to manage your medical needs promptly. Inquire about how this is handled.

10. *Emotional support.* Clearly, this is part of your treatment. Inquire what services are available for supporting you and your family. You'll want to ask about psychological support, as well as financial needs in case issues arise and money is tight due to missing time from work.

Jill's comments:

I originally had my breast cancer treatment 2 years ago at a local hospital. Things went fine. But now that I'm dealing with metastatic disease, I really want to be sure that I am in the best of hands to provide me the optimal treatment for longevity and quality of life. So I went to an NCI designated comprehensive cancer center. I'm being taken care of by an experienced team of doctors and nurses who deal with this kind of situation every day. That gives me great peace of mind.

10. I want to be able to participate in the decision-making about my treatment. How can I do this?

Patients deserve to be empowered so that they can actively participate in decisions about their care and treatment. Some physicians are reluctant to empower women in this way. It is a patient's right and should be a key factor in deciding where she wants to receive her treatment. Seek an oncology team that specializes in breast cancer and has a great deal of experience in treating and managing patients with metastatic disease. The purpose of treating your metastatic breast cancer is to help you live as long as possible with a good quality of life. Since different people have different beliefs and values, it is important that you communicate these to your healthcare team so that everyone can be working for the same goals.

Patients deserve to be empowered so that they can actively participate in decisions about their care and treatment.

Studies show that the more we empower a patient and give her a solid knowledge base about her breast cancer, the more satisfied she is with her care. This includes educating other family members when appropriate. There will be family members who will be helping with your care, so they need to understand the treatment plan and know what to expect.

11. I've heard the term "multidisciplinary care," or "tumor board," used. What is this and should I be requesting this?

A key advantage to having a multidisciplinary team approach is the special expertise each healthcare professional offers to each patient's unique situation. Centers that hold weekly breast cancer case conferences (sometimes referred to as breast cancer tumor boards) to discuss in detail a patient's clinical condition, diagnostic findings, and recommendations for optimal treatment find that these meetings are beneficial to the patient's overall well-being and clinical outcome. Since your case will be discussed in light of the most up-to-date research findings, this is a way that you can ensure that you are being given individualized attention and care by a team of experts. All NCI (National Cancer Institute) accredited cancer centers are required to conduct such conferences on a regular basis and maintain records of the cases presented. Usually the patient is informed by the physician presenting her case that her clinical situation is going to be discussed by the team. The doctor then informs the patient of the discussion and outcome of that presentation, including clinical research trials that you may choose to participate in. Ask your doctor if she is part of a multidisciplinary team and if your case will be presented at their tumor board meeting.

12. Why would I be participating in a clinical trial now? I thought that they were just for women with breast cancer that hadn't spread?

Having as many treatment options available to you as possible can be valuable. Breast centers who participate in clinical trials can usually offer more innovative treatment options. Many clinical trials offer you treatment that is at least as good as the **standard of care** and, possibly, better. If you are asked to participate in such a trial, you are also paving the way for the development of innovative research that will make an important impact on other women diagnosed in the future. You will be closely monitored throughout the treatment process so that data can be collected about your experience with the chemotherapy agents you've been given. (Refer to page 85 regarding clinical trials.)

Standard of care

A diagnostic and treatment process that a clinician should follow for a certain type of patient, illness, or clinical circumstances.

Breast centers who participate in clinical trials can usually offer more innovative treatment options

13. My surgery was done when I was originally diagnosed with breast cancer. Will I still need a breast surgeon to be involved now?

You have probably already had breast cancer surgery done when you were originally diagnosed with breast cancer. There *are* situations, however, that result in needing additional surgery when breast cancer returns. This can be for local control of the disease, diagnostic purposes, or to relieve pain. It is preferable that the surgeon is a **surgical oncologist** who specializes in breast cancer. Such surgeons are often found at a large teaching hospital that is part of a cancer center. There may also be a need for some patients to have a plastic surgeon who specializes in breast reconstruction.

14. How do I select the medical oncologist who will primarily be responsible for my care and treatments?

You will feel more confident being treated by a medical oncologist who specializes in breast cancer. You will want someone who treats a large volume of women with this disease and has access to a spectrum of clinical trials for you to consider. Be sure to also ask how the physician's office practice handles emergency issues, such as a sudden high fever or uncontrolled nausea and vomiting. You will also want to know who will cover for your doctor on weekends or when he or she is on vacation. This doctor should also be a medical oncologist. These are important factors to ask about so that you are confident your case is being well managed.

Ask what education is available to help you prepare for known side effects of treatment. Inquire how patients are referred for wig fittings, as well as any skin care needs that may occur during treatment. Some breast centers offer these services within their facility.

15. Do I need a radiation oncologist?

Most patients who are having breast conservation surgery or have had locally advanced disease have already undergone radiation therapy in some manner. It is valuable to go to a facility that has extensive experience as well as doctors and therapists who specialize in treating this specific type of cancer. They will have a **radiation physicist** on staff who assists with the treatment planning. There are different methods of delivering

Radiation physicist

Makes sure that the equipment is working properly and that the machines deliver the right dose of radiation.

radiation for breast cancer treatment today. Some are part of clinical trials and some are standard of care. Patients will want to know how their heart and lungs will be protected from the radiation field. At some point during your treatment for metastatic disease, you may need radiation therapy to help shrink the tumor(s), provide local control of the disease, or reduce pain symptoms. (Refer to page 29 regarding radiation.)

16. I want to make sure that my doctors are communicating with one another and not relying on me to give them updates. How do I make sure my medical oncologist, radiation oncologist, and family doctor are talking?

You want to know that you are being cared for by a team who stays well connected with you and with each other.

You need to have confidence that you are being watched over and cared for appropriately. Some facilities have nurse practitioners who stay in touch with the patients via telephone once they are home from surgery and/or chemotherapy. More are beginning to offer **patient navigators** to help with coordination of care. The team of professionals taking care of you also needs to stay in close contact with one another. Tumor board conferences (refer to page 17) are another way that your team stays in touch. Ask them how they communicate and keep each other informed about your condition and needs. You want to know that you are being cared for by a team who stays well connected with you and with each other. Feeling confident that you are receiving good continuity of care provides wonderful peace of mind to you and your family.

Patient navigators

An individual who assists patients in navigating their care and treatment by assisting them with scheduling appointments, answering questions related to test results, patient education, support, and providing guidance in decision-making across the continuum of care.

17. Who do I call when I have an emergency or urgent problem?

When an urgent medical problem arises, such as vomiting that won't subside, a clear process needs to be in place for patient management. Ask what the doctor's procedures are for handling such emergencies. A breast center needs to have available a professional healthcare provider 24 hours a day, 7 days a week to handle emergencies. In addition to this, the patients should know how to access this service and know they can confidently rely on it. Though it is hoped that you will not need such services, it's important they are in place and can be readily accessed.

18. The stress of thinking about what may lie ahead is overwhelming to me. Who can help me with these feelings?

You need to be treated as a total person. You are not only a stage IV breast cancer patient. You may be a schoolteacher, recently divorced, with two young children and a mother who has chronic illnesses and lives with you. Breast centers usually provide social work counseling, psychotherapy services, and nurses along with others to help you along this journey. Some offer to match a breast cancer patient with a survivor volunteer based on her age, stage of disease, and anticipated treatment plan, including those with metastatic disease. This isn't always possible but when it is, it provides a unique level of support for someone just embarking on chronic treatment. Patients usually value the opportunity to talk with others. Some breast centers also offer special support groups for women dealing with metastatic disease.

Breast Centers like Johns Hopkins offer special retreats for women with stage IV breast cancer. These events are designed to help patients and their family members as they take the journey together as a family with the treatment of this disease. Such programs, funded by generous donors, can help a patient make decisions regarding continuation of treatment, define quality of life from her perspective and ensure that her voice is heard when it comes to treatment and end of life wishes. There programs are not limited to Johns Hopkins patients. So for more information visit *www.hopkinsbreastcenter.org.*

There are also annual conferences held by the Metastatic Breast Cancer Network. Watch for these educational programs as well and plan to attend if you want to learn more about research endeavors associated with this disease and its treatment as well as to network with others.

PART THREE

Decisions Regarding Surgery and Radiation for Treatment of Metastatic Disease

My cancer has spread to my brain and is located in one spot. What are the treatment options for this type of metastasis?

How is radiation used for treatment or control of metastatic breast cancer?

I've had radiation already to shrink my cancer in the spine and it has regrown. Can I have radiation again?

More . . .

Lumpectomy

Breast cancer surgery to remove the breast cancer and a small amount of normal tissue surrounding it.

Mastectomy

Surgery that removes the whole breast.

If you've been diagnosed with and treated for breast cancer in the past, you more than likely had either a **lumpectomy** or **mastectomy**. If this is your first breast cancer diagnosis, and it was discovered from the onset that it has spread to other organs, then you probably haven't had any surgery. The following is some information related to surgical decisions and what you might expect.

19. I had a lumpectomy and axillary node dissection done 3 years ago and now the cancer has returned to my bones. Will the doctor need to do a mastectomy now?

No, the concern isn't about breast cancer still being in your breast. The surgery or radiation that you had 3 years ago took care of that. The issue now is treating the disease that has spread elsewhere. The time has come for **systemic treatment**, which is treatment that will travel throughout your body no matter where the cancer cells may have gone. Medicines are used to treat disease when it has spread. If you are experiencing bone pain, radiation may also be given to shrink a specific area where a tumor exists that is pressing on nerves causing the pain.

Chrissie's comments:

I was really hoping that the doctor would simply tell me that I can have a mastectomy and some pills to treat my cancer. Having now met with her and understanding my situation better, I realize that doing surgery isn't the first priority; treating the disease where it has spread needs to be my first focus.

20. My cancer has spread to my brain and is located in one spot. What are the treatment options for this type of metastasis?

Sometimes when the cancer is in one specific spot and is relatively small, it can be surgically treated, including when it is found to be in the brain. A neurosurgeon would be consulted about this type of surgical procedure. More than likely, this type of surgery would be followed by radiation to the brain.

Andrea's comments:

Learning my cancer had spread to my brain was devastating. I had been having headaches, something that rarely happens to me. The cancer is in one spot and the doctors said that it could probably be surgically removed. This gives me great hope for the future that I'll be around longer to spend time with my children.

21. I have disease in my liver. Can I get a liver transplant as my treatment?

Unfortunately, no. Liver transplants are more for treatment of disease in the liver that is not cancer related. Medicines are needed to treat cancer that has spread to the liver. When the cancer in the liver is limited to just one small area, there may be other options (refer to page 101).

Sometimes when the cancer is in one specific spot and is relatively small, it can be surgically treated, including when it is found to be in the brain.

22. I haven't had surgery yet of any kind because when my cancer was discovered it was also found to have already spread to my bones. Based on my scans, the cancer is now in control. Will the doctor consider doing breast cancer surgery and radiation now?

When breast cancer is in control or only small amounts of disease have been found in another organ site, more and more women are having breast cancer surgery. The size of the original tumor in the breast determines if a lumpectomy or mastectomy would be most appropriate. This rids the body of the source of the disease and some studies have shown that, when it is possible to do this type of procedure, it may prolong survival. The clinical circumstances have to be very specific, however, so not everyone is a candidate.

Decisions About Radiation to Treat Metastatic Breast Cancer

Radiation is considered local treatment and is designed to treat the area where the radiation is being given. Women who have had a lumpectomy for treatment of their original breast cancer more than likely had radiation of the breast following that surgery, to prevent local recurrence of the breast cancer. Now you are dealing with a different situation. The breast cancer has returned in a distant organ outside of the breast where it first began.

23. How is radiation used for treatment or control of metastatic breast cancer?

In a variety of ways. To shrink the tumors, to control pain caused by the tumors, and, for small tumors, to actually shrink the tumor until it disappears. Cancers that have spread to the bone are sometimes treated this way if they are causing pain and/or are limited to just a few specific spots. Radiation is also used to treat and control brain metastasis.

Emily's comments:

The pain I was having in my back was unbearable for a while until the doctor decided to do radiation. I would never have imagined that doing a couple weeks of daily radiation would have taken nearly all of my back pain away but it did. What a relief to feel more like myself and regain my quality of life.

24. How does the doctor protect the rest of my body from getting radiation it doesn't need?

With the help of 3D imaging, CAT scans, MRIs, and a physicist, the radiation oncology team can plan your radiation so that it targets the specific areas that need treatment. "Blocks" are also created to help protect other vital organs and tissue from receiving radiation. Some tissue may be radiated that is at the edge of the radiation field. The doctor will discuss with you what side effects you may experience, if any, and how long they will last. (Refer to Part 6, regarding side effects.) Radiation in general is well tolerated with the primary side effect being fatigue.

25. I've had radiation already to shrink my cancer in the spine and it has regrown. Can I have radiation again?

Your radiation oncologist needs to carefully review the amount of radiation you have received thus far to determine if you can have more. There is a maximum dosage that it is recommended that you not exceed. Records are kept of the dosages you received for each treatment so that this can be tracked and factored into the decision-making about further radiation if and when it is needed.

PART FOUR

Chemotherapy for Treatment of Metastatic Disease

How will my oncologist decide how much
chemotherapy to give me?

How will the doctors determine if the
chemotherapy is working?

What are my chances of remission,
and how long will it last?

More . . .

26. What is chemotherapy and how does it work?

Chemotherapy ("chemo") is a cancer treat-ment that uses medicines to stop the growth of cancer cells.

Chemotherapy ("chemo") is a cancer treatment that uses medicines to stop the growth of cancer cells. Technically, drugs that kill bacteria and other germs are also called chemotherapy, but the term is most commonly used to refer to cancer-killing drugs.

Although most people think of chemotherapy as intrave-nous infusions, it can also be taken by mouth or injected into a muscle. Because the chemotherapy eventually gets into the bloodstream, all three of these methods of admin-istration allow the chemotherapy to attack cancer cells at sites great distances from the original cancer. Sometimes it is better to place the chemotherapy directly into an organ like the liver, into the spinal fluid, or into a body cavity like the peritoneum (abdominal cavity) or pleura (chest cavity). This is usually done in conjunction with the body-wide (systemic) treatment, but not always.

Chemotherapy drugs work in a variety of ways, but they all work by killing cancer cells or stopping them from grow-ing. Most chemotherapy drugs are not too smart. These cytotoxic drugs work by killing fast-growing cells, but they cannot tell the difference between a cancer cell and a healthy cell. Cancer cells grow much faster than even the fastest growing normal cells. If the cell is unable to reproduce, it will eventually die without another cell to replace it. This results in a decrease in the number of cancer cells. Some normal cells grow very slowly and others, like hair, blood cells, and the cells lining the gastrointestinal tract, grow relatively fast. That is why side effects of chemotherapy may include low blood cell counts, mouth sores, diarrhea, hair loss, and infertility.

Jessica's comments:

Losing my hair again was devastating to me. I was so excited when it grew back before after my chemo. Now it's gone again and I don't know if it will grow back based on all the medicines I'm taking. That may seem like a petty issue to most people but for me seeing my own hair back on my head meant that I was healthy again. So seeing that it is gone and having others know it is gone represents illness that I find very scary. It would be easier for me if the treatments I had didn't cause hair loss. The doctors feel that chemotherapy, however, is my best option right now so I'll do what I have to do to keep fighting off this disease.

27. I got several drugs before, why am I only getting one now?

Chemotherapy works by killing cancer cells. There are a number of ways to do this, and different drugs attack cancer cells in different ways. If a mugger in a dark alley attacked you, you probably would not just hit him in the stomach. You would have a better chance of stopping him if you hit him in several vulnerable spots—stomach, head, back, and groin. When oncologists choose to use several anti-cancer drugs (**combination chemotherapy**) they are doing the biological equivalent of your multi-pronged attack on the mugger.

The downside of this approach is that the combined drugs have more side effects than single drugs. Breast cancer that has not metastasized is potentially curable, and oncologists throw out all the stops to do this, even if there is a chance of more toxicity. Most people are willing to accept the short-term risk of toxicity if there is a reasonable chance that the chemotherapy will cure their

Combination chemotherapy

Treatment using more than one anti-cancer drug at a time.

cancer. Unfortunately, when breast cancer has recurred or spread, it cannot be cured, and there is a need to make big changes in how it is treated. The goal of treatment is no longer cure, but to enjoy life for as long as possible. Since you will likely be getting some form of anti-cancer treatment for the rest of your life, doctors need to balance your quality of life with the side effects that the treatment will cause. For that purpose, single agent chemotherapy is often as effective as combination chemotherapy, and less toxic.

That does not mean that oncologists never use combinations of drugs in treating metastatic breast cancer. Sometimes two or more drugs work together to augment each other's actions with few additional side effects. This is especially true of the newer targeted therapies, which oncologists often combine with a traditional chemotherapy drug to enhance their effect.

28. When I was first diagnosed with breast cancer, I was treated with adjuvant chemotherapy. Will I get the same drugs again?

Micrometastases

Small numbers of cancer cells that have spread from the primary tumor to other parts of the body and are too few to be picked up in a screening or diagnostic test.

When you got adjuvant chemotherapy, the hope was that it would eradicate all of the **micrometastases** that were in your body. Unfortunately, that did not work, and those seeds have now grown into obvious metastases. It does not make any sense to treat your cancer with drugs to which it is already resistant. Therefore, your oncologist will probably want to choose new drugs to fight your cancer. This is especially true if your cancer returned while you were getting those drugs, or shortly after you stopped taking them. If you got adjuvant chemotherapy many years ago, your oncologist may decide to include one or two of those drugs in your new treatment program since they worked so well at the outset. It is possible that they will be more effective when combined with a new agent.

29. How will my oncologist decide how much chemotherapy to give me?

Your oncologist will individualize your chemotherapy dose and schedule to maximize the chance that your cancer will respond and minimize the side effects that you will experience. The initial doses will depend upon your height and weight (body surface area), vital organ function (especially the kidney and liver), and general health status. Your oncologist may need to adjust the dose of chemotherapy in subsequent cycles if you are having unacceptable side effects or need to delay the start of the next treatment.

Your oncologist will decide how many cycles of chemotherapy to give you based on how well your cancer responds to treatment (*efficacy*) and on the side effects (*toxicity*) that you experience. They may give it for a set number of cycles, but, when treating metastatic breast cancer, oncologists usually continue treatment as long as it is working.

30. Do I have to be hospitalized to get my treatments?

Certain types of breast cancer treatment require a short stay in the hospital, but most do not. You will most likely get your chemotherapy in your oncologist's office or in an outpatient clinic. Many cancer patients enjoy the camaraderie and support of others who are getting chemotherapy, but most chemotherapy infusion suites

Your oncologist will individualize your chemotherapy dose and schedule to maximize the chance that your cancer will respond and minimize the side effects that you will experience.

Many cancer patients enjoy the camaraderie and support of others who are getting chemotherapy, but most chemotherapy infusion suites also offer you the option of getting your treatment in a private room.

also offer you the option of getting your treatment in a private room. You should make sure that your doctor has a facility that will meet your needs. It can take anywhere from 1 to 8 or more hours to get your treatment, depending on the type of chemotherapy that you are getting. You will probably get your chemotherapy while seated in a comfortable reclining-type chair. There are beds available in some infusion centers, but you will probably be more comfortable in the specially designed chemotherapy recliners. If there are no TVs at the place where you get chemotherapy, you may want to bring your own DVD player, iPod, or a book to read. You should dress comfortably, and you may want to bring a snack or light lunch. It will probably be possible for a family member or friend to keep you company while you get your treatment, but space is usually quite limited and you may want to nap during much of your infusion. Although there is nothing particularly scary about seeing someone receiving chemotherapy, young children are easily bored and should probably stay at home.

31. How is chemotherapy given?

Oncologists give chemotherapy in different ways, depending on the location of your metastases and the drugs that your oncologist gives you. The four most common methods are: intravenous, oral, intramuscular, and intrathecal.

The *intravenous (IV)* route is the most common way of giving chemotherapy. An oncology nurse inserts a small plastic needle into one of the veins in your lower arm so that the chemotherapy can flow through it. Since a needlestick is required to get into the vein, you may have some temporary, minor discomfort. After that, infusion of the chemotherapy is usually painless. Chemotherapy flows from a plastic bag, through the needle and catheter, into the bloodstream. Sometimes the oncology nurse uses a syringe to push the chemotherapy through the tubing. Chemotherapy can also be infused into your veins through a **vascular access device (VAD)**.

The *oral (po)* route takes the form of a pill, capsule, or liquid taken by mouth. This is the easiest and most convenient method since it can be done at home.

The *intramuscular (im)* method involves getting an injection directly into the muscle. There is a slight pinch as the nurse places the needle into the muscle of the arm, thigh, or buttocks; however, the procedure lasts only a few seconds. This route is usually not used to give breast cancer chemotherapy, but it is used occasionally to give hormonal therapy.

Intrathecal chemotherapy may be necessary when breast cancer spreads to the nervous system. This usually involves injecting chemotherapy directly into the spinal fluid after your doctor does a spinal tap.

32. What are ports and vascular access devices? Do I need one?

Vascular access devices (VADs, central venous catheters, ports) can make it easier and safer for you to get your treatment. They are not always necessary, but, if you are like most chemotherapy patients, once you have one, you will like it. Intravenous chemotherapy and repeated blood draws can make your veins fragile. It often becomes hard for the nurse to find your vein. This can be very stressful and uncomfortable for you. If some chemotherapy drugs leak out of a fragile vein, they can damage your soft tissues.

A VAD is a special thin tube (catheter) placed under the skin and inserted into a large vein in your chest. This is an outpatient procedure. A surgeon or **radiologist** will thread the catheter through a vein in your chest, or sometimes your arm, until it reaches a large vein near the heart. The catheter may be left in place for a number of months or years until it is no longer needed.

Complications are rare, but as with any operation, no matter how minor, complications are possible. These include:

- *Bleeding.* This may occur when the catheter is inserted into the vein.

- *Collapsed lung (pneumothorax).* The risk of a collapsed lung varies with the skill of the person inserting the catheter and the site of placement. It is most likely to happen during placement of a catheter in the chest, although the risk is still small.

- *Infection.* This risk is present for as long as the catheter is in your body. It may require treatment with antibiotics in the hospital or removal of the catheter.

- *Blockage or kinking of the catheter.* A kinked or blocked catheter may need to be repositioned or replaced. Regular flushing of the catheter helps reduce blockage.

- *Pain.* You may experience pain at the place where the catheter is inserted or where it lies under your skin. This usually disappears a few days after the catheter has been in.

- *Shifting of the catheter.* A catheter that has moved out of place can sometimes be repositioned, but if this does not work, it must be replaced.

There are several different types of VADs. They are:

Implantable port—a hollow round disk, about the size of a quarter, is placed under the skin, usually on the chest wall under the collarbone. To access the device, the nurse inserts a special needle through the skin into the port. If this hurts you, she can apply a numbing cream to the skin before she inserts the needle. A nurse must flush the device once a month to prevent it from clotting. No other care is required between treatments. Since this device is completely under the skin, you can shower and bathe with no worries.

Rather than being buried under the skin, the *external catheter* (Hickman or PICC line) tube exits the chest wall, usually under the collarbone. These catheters require frequent flushing and dressings. Your nurse will teach you how to change this dressing and care for the catheter. Since the end of the catheter is exposed, there is a slightly higher risk of infection than with the implantable catheter, and you will need to take special precautions when you shower or bathe. External *PICC lines* (*peripherally inserted central catheter*) are useful for short-term use or as a temporary measure until your doctor can have an implantable port placed. Long-term external catheters (Hickman) are useful when giving chemotherapy continually or in patients who are "needle phobic" and unable to tolerate the needlesticks required to access an implantable port.

In addition to their use in administering chemotherapy, you can get IV fluids, antibiotics, bisphosphonates, and blood products through the VAD. You can usually get blood drawn from the port, so you will be able to avoid frequent needlesticks for blood tests.

33. Do I have a choice of how I want to get my chemotherapy?

Chemotherapy is usually given in your veins, but sometimes it can be taken by mouth or as an intramuscular injection. You usually do not have a choice as to how it is given. Very few chemotherapeutic drugs are available as pills. Your doctor will pick the best chemotherapy for you based on where your cancer metastases are, your overall medical condition, and past treatment. People usually think that pills have fewer side effects than intravenous treatment, but this is not always the case. In fact, it is sometimes easier to control the dose and the side effects of intravenous chemotherapy. The side effects of chemotherapy depend on the properties of the drug, not on how you take it. Today, capecitabine is the most frequently used oral chemotherapeutic agent in treating breast cancer. Your oncologist decides how many pills you should take based on your height and weight. You usually take capecitabine twice a day for 2 weeks of a 3-week cycle, but your doctor may decide some other frequency is better for you.

The side effects of chemotherapy depend on the properties of the drug, not on how you take it.

34. What is a chemotherapy cycle?

Oncologists give chemotherapy according to a particular schedule that is based on the type of cancer being treated and the particular drugs being used. Chemotherapy may be given daily, weekly, every 2 to 3 weeks, or monthly. These treatment days are followed by rest days to allow your body time to recover from the effects of chemotherapy. This schedule of treatment and rest days is a *cycle*. There usually is no choice on the interval or for how many days of the cycle you will receive chemotherapy. Your oncologist will decide how many cycles of chemotherapy to give you based on how well your cancer responds to treatment, and on the side effects that you experience. They may give it for a set number of cycles, but when treating metastatic breast cancer, oncologists usually continue treatment as long as it is working.

35. How will the doctors determine if the chemotherapy is working?

It usually takes two or three cycles of chemotherapy before your oncologist will know if it is working. After two or three cycles, your oncologist will repeat your scans to see if your metastases have gotten bigger or smaller. If there are new metastases or the ones that you have now are bigger, your oncologist will stop the treatment that you are taking, and discuss alternative forms of treatment with you. It does not make any sense to continue with a treatment regimen that is not working. You and your oncologist should be thrilled if the size and number of your metastases are smaller, but you should also be pleased if your cancer has not gotten any worse. Without treatment, metastatic breast cancer progresses, and, after a couple of months, if it is stable, it is probably because the chemotherapy has stopped it from growing. It is quite possible that there will be less cancer the next time your doctor repeats the scans.

"Stable or improved disease" is the definition of success that you and your oncologist should use to assess how well the chemotherapy is working. It sometimes takes a couple of months to see this, and that is why you have to wait before you repeat the scans. However, if it is obvious from your doctor's examination that the cancer is growing at a fast pace, even after one cycle therapy, there is probably no reason to continue it. You or your oncologist might also stop the chemotherapy if you are having unusually severe side effects.

"Stable or improved disease" is the definition of success that you and your oncologist should use to assess how well the chemotherapy is working.

41

It is essential that you understand how your oncologist will determine if the chemotherapy is working. You should know when the doctor will make this assessment, and how. It may not always be necessary to do a scan. If, for example, your doctor can feel an enlarged **lymph node** in your neck, she will measure this with a ruler each time you come for a visit. If you have cancer in your liver, your liver blood tests may be elevated, and your doctor can follow these to know if you are responding to treatment. Even in these situations, your oncologist will probably want to repeat scans from time to time, so that she can more fully assess your response to chemotherapy.

In addition to measuring the amount and size of your metastases, your oncologist may also use your symptoms to know if the chemotherapy is working. If the chemotherapy makes you feel better, this is usually a sign that it is working. Good clinical signs that the chemotherapy is working include pain that improves with chemotherapy, a poor appetite or weight loss that is now better, or feeling less tired.

In summary, the definition of "working" is when the cancer is not getting any worse. Oncologists generally continue giving chemotherapy as long as it is working, or until you have unacceptable side effects. You should expect your doctor to assess this every two to three cycles of chemotherapy. Sometimes this assessment is spread out a bit after you have had more chemotherapy.

Lymph nodes

Tissues in the lymphatic system that filter lymph fluid and help the immune system fight disease.

36. What kind of newer therapies are available for women with metastatic disease who have already had most of the chemotherapy drugs you have mentioned and the cancer continues to grow?

This is certainly a major concern for patients and their families—seeing the disease progress despite receiving powerful chemotherapy drugs. There are new therapies that, as a result of clinical trial results, have demonstrated a survival benefit for patients when other chemo drugs have failed to work. An example of a new drug recently approved by the FDA is eribulin mesylate (Halaven). This drug was tested as part of a research study called EMBRACE. It was compared against other single use chemotherapy drugs, targeted biologic therapy, or hormonal therapy as selected by the medical oncologist. The results showed that women taking this drug survived several months longer than those on a different single agent treatment regimen. Such research continues to be ongoing so that more treatment options and better treatment methods can be provided for women in the future.

37. My doctor just told me that my cancer is in remission. Does that mean that I'm cured?

Remission is the word that oncologists use to describe how well the anti-cancer treatment is working. It is not the same as *cure*. Remissions are *complete* or *partial*. Complete remission means that there is no longer any sign of cancer on your examination, blood work, or scans. *Partial remission* means that there is less cancer in your body than there was before treatment, but that there is still some sign of cancer on your examination, blood work, or scans. Sometimes *partial remissions* become *complete remissions* after you get more treatment. The more cancer the treatment kills the better, and complete remissions usually last longer than partial remissions. Unfortunately, when it comes to metastatic breast cancer, even complete remissions are not forever. Though not curable, metastatic breast cancer is usually quite responsive to initial therapy, and there is a good chance that you will enjoy a remission for some time before the cancer grows back.

38. What are my chances of remission, and how long will it last?

The likelihood that your cancer will respond to treatment depends on many complex factors.

That is not an easy question to answer. Some women with metastatic breast cancer live with their disease in remission for years, while others never have a remission and die within months. The likelihood that your cancer will respond to treatment depends on many complex factors. Your overall health and well-being and the amount of metastatic disease are important, but the most important predictor is how well you respond to the first couple of cycles of therapy. Usually, the faster and more complete your initial response, the fuller and longer it will last. Every time your breast cancer comes back, the chance of it responding to a new treatment regimen decreases and the duration of the remission gets a bit shorter. With time, your breast cancer will no longer respond to treatment and the focus of your care will change to managing the symptoms, often with the help of palliative care or hospice nurses. Although the proper time for this transition is a very personal decision, most oncologists feel that the chances of responding to additional chemotherapy are virtually nonexistent if you have not responded to your last three chemotherapy regimens, or if you are spending most of your day in bed or a chair.

Breast cancer that has metastasized to the bone or soft tissues generally grows more slowly, and responds to treatment more completely and longer, than breast cancer that involves the liver, lung, or brain. Breast cancer that recurs after many years generally grows more slowly and responds to treatment better than breast cancer that recurs during, or shortly after, the initial diagnosis and treatment.

39. I feel pretty good during my chemotherapy treatments, and I worry that the treatment isn't strong enough. Is it more likely to work if I get more severe side effects?

This is a common myth. There is really no link between how well the chemotherapy works and the severity of the side effects. Different people tolerate chemotherapy in different ways, and some chemotherapy drugs cause more side effects than others do. If you are not having severe side effects from your treatment, relax and don't worry. There are now excellent medicines that prevent many of the side effects of chemotherapy. You should take these as prescribed and without fear.

There is really no link between how well the chemotherapy works, and the severity of the side effects.

40. How often will I see my oncologist during my chemotherapy treatments?

You will see your oncologist regularly throughout your treatment. At these visits, your doctor will see how you are tolerating the treatment and if you are having side effects. He will order medication to relieve any side effects, and, if these are severe, he may adjust your treatment schedule or dose. Another reason for these visits is so that your oncologist can see if your cancer is responding to the treatment.

Your oncologist will probably want to see you at the beginning of each cycle of chemotherapy. Most oncologists try to do this the same day that you get the chemotherapy, but sometimes it is more convenient to do this a day or two before. If you have any problems in the middle of your chemotherapy cycle, you should call your doctor to see if she wants to see you sooner. If your oncologist works with a nurse practitioner or physician's assistant, she may see you at some of these visits. The primary reason for these scheduled visits is to be certain that it is safe to begin the next cycle of chemotherapy. You will have blood drawn to be sure that your blood counts have returned to normal. Your doctor will examine you and ask questions about any side effects of chemotherapy that you had during the last cycle of chemotherapy. You can help your doctor by keeping a diary of any problems, concerns, or questions that you had during the last cycle of chemotherapy. When it is time to see how well your cancer is responding to the chemotherapy, your oncologist will have you get the necessary scans and blood work a few days before your visit. He will review these with you at your visit and discuss future chemotherapy plans with you.

41. Since the chemotherapy affects my immune system, is it still okay for me to work while taking it? Are there any precautions I should use in the work place or in other social settings?

The purpose of chemotherapy is to allow you to live your life in as normal a manner as possible, for as long as possible. The chemotherapy will certainly affect you, but you should strive to go about your regular business as much as you can. Though the chemotherapy will affect your immune system, this is really only a problem when your white blood cell count is low.

White blood cells (WBC), more specifically, the group of white blood cells called neutrophils fight infection, and, when they are low, you are at increased risk for infection. Your white blood cells drop to their lowest point (**nadir**) in the middle of your cycle of chemotherapy, stay there for a few days, and then gradually increase back to normal. Your greatest risk of infection is, therefore, in the middle of your chemotherapy cycle.

It is prudent to minimize your exposure to sources of infections during the entire time that you are on chemotherapy, but this is most important during the nadir period. You do not need to be a hermit during this period, but you should not go out of your way to be around people with colds and fevers. This is easy to do in your own home where you can ask visitors to stay away if they are sick.

This is harder to do at work or in large social settings, especially if you do not want to share your diagnosis with co-workers and friends. You need to be in control of your

The purpose of chemotherapy is to allow you to live your life in as normal a manner as possible, for as long as possible.

Nadir

The low point of blood counts that occurs as a result of chemotherapy.

environment, especially when your WBC count is low. If this is not possible, it is best to avoid these situations all together or, if you must, limit the time of your exposure and wear a mask. It should go without saying that you should not share things like towels or drinking glasses, and always use common sense hygiene measures.

Actually, most infections that people get during chemotherapy come from the germs that normally inhabit your intestinal tract or skin

Actually, most infections that people get during chemotherapy come from the germs that normally inhabit your intestinal tract or skin. Your immune system usually keeps these germs in their own place, but when your WBC count is low, they can sneak through these natural defenses and cause an infection. Over the years, studies have shown that antibiotics, nutritional supplements, or a change in your diet will not prevent this from happening. Fortunately, the majority of patients who get chemotherapy do not get infected, and those that do usually respond to antibiotics quite nicely. However, immediate treatment is critical, and it is very important for you to call your doctor right away if you have a fever or any signs or symptoms of infection—even if these occur at 2:00 in the morning!

42. My doctor checks my blood count just before I get my next dose of chemotherapy. Why does he also need to check it 1–2 weeks later?

Your blood counts reach their nadir about 1–2 weeks after you get your chemotherapy. After a few days, they start to rise, and usually return to normal in time for you to start your next cycle of chemotherapy. Your doctor checks your blood counts on the day that you get chemotherapy (or the day before) so that he will know if it safe for you to start your next cycle of chemotherapy. If your white blood cells or **platelets** are too low, you will probably need to wait until they return to a safe

Platelets

Components of blood that assist in clotting and wound healing.

level before you get your next treatment. Your oncologist may also want to know how low your counts get at their nadir. This helps her decide if she needs to modify the dose of your chemotherapy or the interval between your treatments. If your WBC nadir is unusually low, or if you have **neutropenic fever** or infection, your oncologist may decide to give you a cytokine (Neulasta or Neupogen) the day after your next chemotherapy infusion, to try to prevent this from happening again. He also uses these mid-cycle nadir blood counts to advise you on the need for any special precautions or treatments to protect yourself from infection (due to low WBC counts) or bleeding (due to low platelet counts).

Neutropenic fever

A fever due to a low white blood cell count, usually caused by a side effect of chemotherapy.

43. Is there anything that I can do to bring my blood counts up?

Not really. Your bone marrow makes your blood cells, and it is particularly sensitive to chemotherapy. Chemotherapy causes some degree of bone marrow suppression in almost everybody. Some chemotherapy drugs are harder on the bone marrow than others, but with time, your blood counts will rise. If your blood counts continue to be low, your doctor may need to decrease the dose of chemotherapy that you are getting. A lower dose of chemotherapy will probably kill fewer cells and allow you to get chemotherapy on schedule. Another approach is for your doctor to give you a cytokine (for example G-CSF, Neupogen, or Neulasta) injection the day after you get your chemotherapy. An oncology nurse usually gives you this injection subcutaneously, or under the skin.

If you are curious about the physiology of how this works, cytokines or colony-stimulating factors (CSFs) are growth factors that stimulate your bone marrow to make white blood cells. CSFs increase the recovery rate from bone marrow side effects of chemotherapy and radiation. Bone marrow side effects lower blood counts. Sometimes oncologists give CSFs in the middle of a chemotherapy cycle to limit the period of neutropenia, especially if you have a severe infection. You may experience some bone discomfort a day or two after you get a CSF. This is due to the rapid growth of blood cells in the confined space of the bone marrow. This pain is usually mild and controlled with acetaminophen (Tylenol) or ibuprofen, but sometimes you have to take stronger medicine for a few days.

44. When I have a problem, should I call my primary care doctor or my oncologist?

That depends on what the problem is. Your cancer or treatment may affect your other medical problems, and it is critical that all of your doctors communicate with each other. For example, the corticosteroids (prednisone or Decadron) that oncologists use as chemotherapy pre-medication, or to help control nausea and vomiting, may make gastric acid problems worse or increase your blood sugar making your diabetes worse. If you have high blood pressure, your doctor may need to adjust your antihypertensive medicines. Most oncologists prefer that your **primary care doctor** continue to manage your non–cancer-related problems, but since your primary care doctor may not always be aware of some of the problems associated with certain cancers or cancer treatments, it is important that you tell your oncologist about all of your medical problems. For example, the low-grade fever and sore throat that your primary doctor usually tells you to treat with acetaminophen and salt water gargles may

Primary care doctor

The physician (internist or family doctor) who takes care of your general healthcare needs.

require hospitalization and intravenous antibiotics in the setting of a chemotherapy-induced low white blood count. A good rule of thumb is, when in doubt, call your oncologist's office, and let them decide who should take care of the problem.

45. Why do I need intrathecal chemotherapy?

Chemotherapy reaches cancer metastases through the bloodstream, but the **blood-brain barrier** interferes with its ability to reach brain metastases. This barrier prevents germs and other disease-causing agents from reaching the brain. The same barrier that prevents germs from reaching the brain and protects you from infections also prevents chemotherapy from reaching your brain and protects brain metastases from chemotherapy. It is very difficult to break down this barrier. The only effective way to get chemotherapy into the brain or the tissues surrounding it (meninges) is to bypass it. Doctors do this by putting the chemotherapy directly into the fluid that surrounds the brain. From there, it can penetrate the cancer cells that seed the lining of the brain (*carcinomatous meningitis*). The fluid that is in contact with the meninges of the brain also circulates down the spinal canal. Therefore, it is possible for your doctor to treat these metastases by doing a spinal tap and injecting chemotherapy into the spinal canal. If you need repeated injections of chemotherapy, it is usually easier to do this through an Ommaya reservoir placed directly into one of the ventricles (lakes of spinal fluid) in your brain. This may sound dangerous, but it really is not. This relatively minor surgical procedure is quite similar to having a port placed in the large veins in your chest.

Blood-brain barrier

A special layer that protects the brain from infection. This layer is made up of a network of blood vessels with thick walls.

46. Is it true that bone marrow transplant is better than standard chemotherapy?

High-dose chemotherapy with bone marrow (or stem cell) transplant is a way of giving high doses of chemotherapy and replacing blood-forming bone marrow cells destroyed by the cancer treatment. It is actually more like a fancy blood transfusion than an organ transplant. Stem cells are removed from the blood or bone marrow of the patient or a donor and are frozen and stored. After the chemotherapy is completed, these stem cells are thawed and given back to the patient through an intravenous infusion. These re-infused stem cells home to the bone marrow where they grow into and restore the body's blood cells.

Though high-dose chemotherapy followed by stem cell transplant is useful in a number of cancers, studies have clearly shown that it does not work any better than standard chemotherapy in the treatment of breast cancer. Indeed, these studies showed that more breast cancer patients died of treatment side effects with this treatment than those who got standard treatment.

47. Is it safe to travel while I am getting chemotherapy?

Although sticking to the chemotherapy schedule is important, the schedule is not nearly as inflexible as many people think that it is. You will probably be getting chemotherapy for the rest of your life. Since the goal of chemotherapy is to allow you to live your life, it is imperative that you do so, sometimes despite the chemotherapy itself. Holidays, vacations, and family life-cycle events are part of everyone's life. Just because you

Since the goal of chemotherapy is to allow you to live your life, it is imperative that you do so, sometimes despite the chemotherapy itself.

are getting chemotherapy does not mean that you need to forgo these pleasures. Tell your oncologist when they will occur, and do not be surprised when she accommodates your chemotherapy schedule around those events. Unless it becomes a regular practice, a day here or there, or an occasional extra week between cycles, will have little impact on how well the chemotherapy works; especially once you have a few treatment cycles under your belt. During your regular cycle of therapy, there are better times to travel than others. The best time to travel is once you are through the period of nadir cytopenias, just before you are due to get your next treatment. Make sure that your oncologist knows of your travel plans, and be sure to carry with you a summary of your chemotherapy treatment and latest blood counts. If you do not have access to a doctor through the friends or relatives whom you plan to visit, ask your oncologist to give you the name of a local oncologist in case you run into trouble. Of course, make sure that you take your oncologist's telephone and fax number with you.

PART FIVE

Hormonal Therapy

How does the doctor determine if I should get
hormonal therapy instead of chemotherapy?

Are there different types of hormonal therapies?
How does my doctor decide which to use?

I am taking hormonal therapy for treatment of my
metastatic breast cancer. I thought chemotherapy
was "better" than hormonal therapy since it is given
intravenously. Is that true or a myth?

More . . .

48. How does the doctor determine if I should get hormonal therapy instead of chemotherapy?

Hormonal therapy is only an option if your cancer cells have hormone receptors present. When your breast cancer was first biopsied, the pathologists tested your cancer cells to see if estrogen receptors (ER) or progesterone receptors (PR) were present. Unless this test found at least one of these hormone receptors, your cancer will not respond to hormone therapy. Breast cancers may keep the same hormonal receptor profile forever. However, from time to time, hormone receptor–positive cancers become negative. It is unusual for a hormone receptor–negative cancer to change to hormone receptor–positive. If your doctor suspects that the hormone receptor status of your cancer may have changed, she may want to biopsy one of the metastatic spots and send it to a laboratory for estrogen and progesterone receptor tests.

If your cancer is not estrogen receptor–positive or progesterone receptor–positive or both, chemotherapy is your only option. If it is hormone receptor–positive, your doctor can use either chemotherapy or hormonal therapy to treat your cancer.

Hormone therapy is usually the first treatment used in postmenopausal women, unless their tumor is hormone receptor negative. Hormone therapy is especially useful in patients whose metastatic disease involves only bone or soft tissue. Though it is also useful in treating metastases to the vital organs (liver, lung, etc.), chemotherapy often works faster in these situations.

If your cancer has recurred while you are taking adjuvant hormonal therapy, your doctor may prefer to switch to chemotherapy as the initial treatment for your metastatic cancer, especially if your cancer involves sites other than the bone or soft tissues. Another option would be to switch to a different type of hormonal therapy than you are currently using.

Chrissie's comments:

It frustrates me that I'm only receiving hormonal therapy right now for treatment of my recently discovered metastatic disease. I want it cut out, killed with chemo, and zapped away with radiation. That makes sense to me. The doctors say that less aggressive treatment may get it into control—that is the mission now. I still think that the mission is to be cured. I need to start thinking of this disease as a chronic disease and that is hard to do.

49. Are there different types of hormonal therapies? How does my doctor decide which to use?

Different types of hormonal therapies are used to treat cancer in postmenopausal women than those used in premenopausal women. Aromatase inhibitors (AIs) are usually the hormonal therapy drug of choice in postmenopausal women. Though tamoxifen is quite effective in postmenopausal women, the AIs work better and have fewer side effects. Because they have no effect on estrogens produced by the ovaries, AIs do not work in premenopausal women.

Sometimes doctors combine hormone therapy (for example, buserelin and tamoxifen). Women whose tumors are hormone receptor positive and have received anti-estrogens

Different types of hormonal therapies are used to treat cancer in postmenopausal women than those used in premenopausal women.

within the past year may still respond to second-line hormonal therapy. Examples of second-line hormonal therapy in postmenopausal women include AIs like anastrozole, letrozole, or exemestane. Fulvestrant is a type of hormonal therapy medicine used to treat post-menopausal women diagnosed with advanced-stage hormone receptor–positive breast cancer. Previous research studies had shown that tamoxifen, anastrozole, letrozole, and exemestane worked similarly in slowing or stopping the growth of metastatic breast cancer cells. More recently a research study was completed administering a higher dose of fulvestrant (going from 250 mg to 500 mg) and shown to be more effective in slowing or stopping the growth of metastatic breast cancer. Premenopausal women with hormone receptor–positive breast cancers should undergo oophorectomy, either surgically, induced with radiation therapy, or with medicine. Tamoxifen is also an option for premenopausal women, whose cancer is hormone receptor–positive and was not treated with it in the past.

50. I have osteoporosis. Is it safe to take an aromatase inhibitor?

Although AIs (anastrozole, letrozole, and exemestane) are usually the hormonal treatments of choice in postmenopausal women with metastatic breast cancer, they may cause problems for women with osteoporosis such as worsening bone loss and increased fracture risk. Fulvestrant binds to the estrogen receptor site in competition with estrogen in the body. Once it binds to the site it can cause the receptor to breakdown, thereby inhibiting normal cellular response to estrogen. It has no agonist effects however, which means that it may not have the same side effects as other hormonal therapy drugs that are part of the aromatase inhibitor drug group. Yet, having osteoporosis does not mean that a woman cannot use an AI. Rather, these women do need to have their osteoporosis managed aggressively and followed closely.

All women should have a bone density study (DEXA scan) before starting an AI. If you are not already doing so, you should take appropriate calcium and vitamin D3 supplements. If you have been taking these supplements regularly, and your bone density scan shows significant **osteopenia** or osteoporosis, you should start taking oral bisphosphonates, such as alendronate sodium (Fosamax), risedronate sodium (Actonel), or ibandronate sodium (Boniva). If you have only osteopenia and have not been taking calcium and vitamin D3, it is reasonable to try these supplements first. By following your bone density on repeated DEXA scans, your doctor can see if these oral therapies are working. Most insurance companies will pay for only one DEXA scan a year; this is usually adequate in this situation.

Osteopenia

A condition of less bone density or bone mass than would be normally expected if you compare a woman to a woman or population of women her age. It is the bone loss that, if it continues, can lead to osteoporosis.

If these measures do not work, intravenous bisphosphonates, such as zoledronic acid (Zometa) given two to three times per year, may allow you to remain on an AI. On the other hand, if you have no major risk factors like blood clots, you and your doctor may want to consider switching to tamoxifen. It is still an excellent drug for breast cancer and it has less risk of aggravating your osteoporosis. If you are prone to falling or have already had a broken bone due to osteoporosis, you should probably simply avoid the AIs altogether.

51. I am taking hormonal therapy for treatment of my metastatic breast cancer. Is it true that chemotherapy is better than hormonal therapy since it is given intravenously?

Many cancer patients make the mistake of thinking that medicine given in the veins is more powerful than medicine given by mouth.

No; hormonal therapy is usually given by mouth or IM injection and it has fewer side effects than most intravenous chemotherapies. Many cancer patients make the mistake of thinking that medicine given in the veins is more powerful than medicine given by mouth. This is not true. It does not really matter how the anti-cancer medicine gets into your body, as long as it does. Some medicines are not absorbed into the bloodstream through the gastrointestinal tract, so doctors have to administer it directly into the bloodstream through a vein. Another common misconception about cancer therapy is to assume that the severity of its side effects is directly related to its anti-tumor strength. Just because a treatment is toxic does not mean that it is effective, and the lack of toxicity does not correlate with inactivity. Unfortunately, many cancer treatments are associated with debilitating side effects, but their anti-cancer effect relates to how the cancer cells respond to the drug, not how it affects your normal cells. Hormonal therapy can actually be more effective than intravenous chemotherapy in a woman whose tumor expresses hormone (estrogen or progesterone) receptors, especially when her metastatic disease is confined to the bones or soft tissue.

PART SIX

Side Effects of Metastatic Breast Cancer and Its Treatment and How to Control Them

What kind of side effects might I expect to experience as a result of getting treatment for my metastatic breast cancer?

My chemotherapy and hormonal therapy have caused me to develop symptoms of menopause. How can I manage these symptoms and feel more like myself again?

I am feeling more joint pain and backaches that make it difficult to walk around. What can I do to manage my pain?

More . . .

52. What kind of side effects might I expect to experience as a result of getting treatment for my metastatic breast cancer?

There are various side effects that a patient may experience while receiving treatment for metastatic disease as well as symptoms of progression of disease that warrant discussion with your doctor. Some are easily controlled and some may be more difficult. No two patients are alike so don't assume if you knew someone with metastatic disease in the past that your situation will mirror theirs. In Questions 52–71, we explain some of the more common side effects. You should discuss these with your oncology team so you know what to expect in relationship to the status of your metastatic disease and the treatment recommendations they are making on your behalf. These questions are not intended to alarm you but to provide you with a comprehensive list of possible issues that may need to be addressed while undergoing treatment.

Marissa's comments:

The side effects from chemo and hormonal therapy were really getting to me. My most miserable problem was night sweats that prevented me from sleeping well. I found that installing a ceiling fan above my bed and keeping it on low all night really helped. Wearing cotton short sleeve and sleeveless nightgowns instead of pajamas that were long sleeved with long pants has been a godsend too. I even found a thing called a "chillow pillow" online that keeps my head feeling cool all night. This makes dealing with these symptoms from treatment a lot more tolerable and doable long term now.

Jill's comments:

I attended a support group provided by the hospital where I'm receiving my treatments. It is for breast cancer survivors but most of the women who were attending were diagnosed early and were completing treatment or had finished treatment long ago. They were fussing and moaning about their hair growing back slowly, or having hot flashes still. This group was not for me and I told the social worker who was the facilitator so. I finally found a group that was specifically for women with metastatic breast cancer. We are all in the same situation— some with disease that is very advanced and others with disease that is more stable but the bottom line is we share the same worries, fears, and hopes. I can relate to these women.

53. Why do I feel so tired most of the time?

Anemia is a common problem for many dealing with cancer. It is especially an issue for those undergoing chemotherapy. By definition, anemia is an abnormally low level of **red blood cells (RBCs)**. These cells contain **hemoglobin**, which provides oxygen to all parts of the body. If RBC levels are low, parts of the body may not be receiving all the oxygen they need to work and function well. In general, people with anemia commonly report feeling tired. The fatigue that is associated with anemia can seriously affect quality of life for some patients and make it difficult for patients to cope at times.

Medications such as epoetin (Procrit, Epogen) or darbepoetin (Aranesp) may be recommended to stimulate your bone marrow to make more red blood cells, raising your blood cell count and increasing your energy level. Such a medication is given by injection under the skin using a

Red blood cells (RBCs)

Cells in the blood with the primary function of carrying oxygen to tissues.

Hemoglobin

The part of the red blood cell that carries the oxygen.

The fatigue that is associated with anemia can seriously affect quality of life for some patients and make it difficult for patients to cope at times.

very small thin needle. The doses vary and it is common to be given one of these medications for this side effect once a week. You might be advised to also take an oral iron supplement while getting these injections.

54. I've heard that some chemotherapy drugs can damage the heart. Is this true?

There are several drugs that can produce a side effect of heart problems: Doxorubicin (Adriamycin), which is a chemotherapy agent, and trastuzumab (Herceptin), which is a biological targeted agent. Your doctor will use a **MUGA** scan or an echocardiogram (**ECHO**) to help determine if it is safe to give these medications. The MUGA or ECHO may be repeated every few months to re-evaluate the heart function and ensure that all is well and that it is safe to continue with your treatment. Congestive heart failure, a weakness of the heart muscle, can occur but is not common. These risks are greater when Herceptin or Adriamycin are given together. Some women are given Herceptin alone with a very low risk to their heart.

MUGA test

A special heart X-ray that determines the strength of the heart.

ECHO test

A special test using ultrasound that determines the strength of the heart.

55. It seems harder to remember things, especially doing math or trying to recall where I put my keys. What is causing these symptoms?

Some refer to this as "chemo brain." People dealing with cancer who are getting chemotherapy as part of their treatment can have trouble remembering names, places, and events or have trouble with concentration or arithmetic. Currently scientific studies are being done to better understand what is causing it and how to counteract it. If you are finding that these symptoms are pretty severe and impacting your ability to function well, ask your family to assist you with the things that are difficult. Make a list of things you need to do and mark each item off as you do it. Keep your keys in the same place so they are easier to find. Most importantly, get your family members to assist you with medication management. A pill box that has the times of day to take your medications is a good idea rather than relying on your memory that you took your medications out of the prescription bottle when they were due. Be sure to tell your doctor if you are having symptoms of chemo brain. Sometimes these same symptoms can be a sign of metastatic cancer cells in the brain, drug side effects, or other causes.

56. Where did my energy go, and what can I do to get it back?

Feeling exhausted or extremely tired is probably the most common side effect patients report. This can happen as a side effect of chemotherapy and/or radiation therapy. Approximately 70 percent of patients with advanced cancers report this as a chronic frustrating symptom. Fatigue can also be triggered by anemia. If there are specific problems you are experiencing that are related to fatigue, such as difficulty sleeping, make your doctor aware so that he might prescribe something for you to help. Ask about how to better manage your pain, if that is a contributing factor. Also ask about coping with your emotional distress, which can increase fatigue. Conserving your energy is important so you are spending your time doing things that are important to you. Make a list of the activities and chores you are trying to accomplish and see about recruiting family and friends to assist you. You may also notice that your energy is better during certain times of the day. The Oncology Nursing Society has a website that provides some specific recommendations related to this side effect. Take a look at *www.cancersymptoms.org/symptoms/fatigue/*. Also visit the National Comprehensive Cancer Network's website for more information at *www.nccn.org*.

57. I've been in treatment for my metastatic breast cancer that spread to my lungs. Lately I've noticed it is getting harder to breathe. What might this be?

Fluid around the lungs, or pleural effusion, is a condition that presents commonly as shortness of breath, dry cough, heaviness feeling in the chest, inability to exercise, and a feeling of not being able to take a deep breath. This is due to extra fluid building up around the pleural spaces of the lungs. A malignant pleural effusion is caused by cancer cells that grow into the **pleural cavity**. Many patients with metastatic breast cancer develop this problem. The diagnosis of pleural effusion is made by physical examination and chest X-ray. Treatment is based on the amount of fluid in your chest and if you have any symptoms. If the fluid collection is considered to be large and given your noticeable symptoms, the doctor may decide to insert a needle through the ribs into the pleural space and remove the fluid. Sometimes this is done with the help and guidance of ultrasound. This procedure is called a **thoracentesis**. It can be done on an outpatient basis. Sometimes the fluid comes back and you will need to have it drained again. If this happens frequently, your doctor may suggest a procedure called **pleurodesis**. Sitting up and

Pleural cavity

A space between the outside of the lungs and the inside wall of the chest.

Thoracentesis

The removal of fluid from the pleural cavity through a hollow needle inserted between the ribs.

Pleurodesis

A procedure that gets rid of the open space between the lung and the chest cavity. This is done to stop fluid from building up in this space. When cancer cells are growing in this space, they make fluid that can collect and cause difficulty breathing. During this surgery, a chemical is placed in the space. Your body's reaction to the chemical causes the lining around the lung to stick to the inside lining of the chest wall.

using pillows for support can make breathing sometimes easier. Reclining chairs may be more helpful for sleeping than trying to lie flat in bed. Oxygen may be given as well to help with breathing. If oxygen is given at home, great care must be taken. The use of matches, cigarettes, or candles is not allowed in the room where the oxygen is in use or being stored. Oxygen containers should be kept far away from gas or electrical heating elements, too. The respiratory therapist or company that provides the oxygen will review other safety measures with you and your family or caregivers.

58. What is lymphedema and how can I manage it if I develop it?

Lymphedema is an abnormal collection of **lymph** fluid in the arms or legs. Lymphatic fluid is in our bodies to fight infection and cancer. When lymph nodes in relatively large numbers have been surgically removed or radiated, however, the pathway for lymphatic drainage can become disrupted and fluid that is sent down the arm, for example, may have trouble returning back up the arm. This results in the arm swelling and staying swollen. Infection, trauma to the arm, or other factors may trigger the lymphedema. Lymphedema can cause discomfort, pain, and limit the use of your arm. Most patients do not develop lymphedema from having nodes removed or having radiation to the armpit area. The incidence of lymphedema is lower in the last 15 years because of improvements in surgical and radiation therapy techniques. If you develop lymphedema you may experience heaviness, throbbing pain or soreness, or a feeling of tightness from your wristwatch, rings, or clothing.

Lymphedema

A condition in which lymph fluid collects in tissues following removal of, or damage to, lymph nodes during surgery, causing the limb or area of the body affected to swell.

Lymph

Fluid carried through the body by the lymphatic system, composed primarily of white blood cells and diluted plasma.

Some prevention steps you can take to help reduce the risk of developing lymphedema include the following:

Perform gentle strengthening and stretching exercises to keep the affected arm working normally.

Avoid lifting or moving heavy objects using that arm after surgery.

Keep skin clean and moisturized, avoid cuts or cracks in the skin, and avoid insect bites whenever possible.

Avoid getting any needlesticks in that arm—such as IVs, vaccinations, or blood draws from the arm where lymph nodes were surgically removed or radiated.

Avoid getting blood pressures taken in that arm too.

Report signs of infection to your doctor right away. If you do get a cut or injury to this arm, wash the cut immediately and apply over-the-counter antibiotic ointment right away.

Report any changes you notice to this arm, such as swelling or feeling of heaviness.

If you develop lymphedema, there are several things that may be helpful. You can elevate the arm, use a compression sleeve, have a massage by a rehabilitation therapist who specializes in lymphedema management, use compression bandaging, or use a pressure pump. For more information about lymphedema, contact the National Lymphedema Network at 800-541-3259 or visit their website at *www.lymphnet.org*.

59. What can I do to manage hair loss?

The technical term for hair loss is alopecia. The hair on your head falls out, and if hair on other parts of your body grows rapidly, it may fall out too (such as eyelashes or eyebrows). Alopecia is a relatively common side effect of several chemotherapy agents used to treat and manage breast cancer. You may have already experienced this when you had your initial breast cancer treatment. For women needing radiation to their brain, hair loss can happen again and may occur in a few areas or all over, depending on how the radiation was given. Hair loss has become a signal that the person is a cancer patient. It can be psychologically and physically difficult to cope with hair loss since it is associated with our self-image, womanliness, health status, and other personal issues related to how we feel about our hair. Getting a wig in advance of hair loss can be helpful so that your hair style, texture, and color can be matched well for you. Some insurance companies cover the expense of a wig. Check your policy and see if your insurance company covers "skull prosthesis for side effects of cancer treatment." Costs that are not covered are tax deductible. There are programs like "Look Good, Feel Good" that most cancer centers offer to their patients. This is a special program available free of charge to show you how to wear turbans, scarves, and makeup to reduce the obvious appearance of hair loss. Ask your doctor or nurse when they are offering this program at the facility where you are getting your treatment.

Alopecia is a relatively common side effect of several chemotherapy agents used to treat and manage breast cancer.

60. My doctor mentioned that he would check my calcium levels periodically. What is this for?

Hypercalcemia is an unusually high level of calcium found in the blood. There are situations in which it can be life threatening, and it is usually associated with a problem with metabolism caused by the cancer. It occurs in 10 to 20 percent of people with cancer. Symptoms that would trigger your doctor to check your blood

Hypercalcemia
Accelerated loss of calcium in bones, leading to elevated levels of the mineral in the bloodstream with symptoms such as nausea and confusion.

level for this side effect include: loss of appetite, nausea, weakness, frequent urination, excessive thirst, feeling confused and unable to concentrate, abdominal pain, or constipation. If the calcium level is very high, it can trigger irregular heartbeat, kidney stones, and loss of consciousness and coma. Intravenous bisphosphonates (zoledronic acid or pamidronate) medications help control this side effect (refer to page 77).

61. It seems harder to fight off colds and flu viruses than it did before. How come?

When harmful bacteria, viruses, or fungi enter the body and the body is not able to fight back to destroy these cells on its own using the immune system, an infection brews. Breast cancer patients are at higher risk of developing an infection because the cancer present in their bodies, along with the treatments being given can weaken their immune systems. Spiking a high fever; chills; sweating; sore throat; mouth sores; pain or burning during urination; diarrhea; shortness of breath; a productive cough; or swelling, redness, or pain around an incision or wound are all symptoms that an infection may be present. To help reduce risk of infection, stay away from young children who may be carriers of flu viruses, colds, and other respiratory illnesses. Though they can look relatively healthy, young children may be harboring germs. This doesn't mean to abandon seeing your children or grandchildren though. It does mean to evaluate how the child is feeling and if he/she has any symptoms (runny nose, fever, cough), that would signal to you that this isn't a good day to have the child sitting on your lap. Family members who live with you or you see frequently should get flu vaccinations too to help reduce the risk of unknowingly bringing viruses your

Breast cancer patients are at higher risk of developing an infection because the cancer present in their bodies, along with the treatments being given, can weaken their immune systems.

way. At the first sign you may be getting an infection (fever, cold, etc.), notify your doctor so he can prescribe something for you.

62. My chemotherapy and hormonal therapy have caused me to develop symptoms of menopause. How can I manage these symptoms and feel more like myself again?

Approximately 40 percent of women dealing with breast cancer develop menopausal symptoms due to breast cancer treatments. This can be particularly an issue for women who are premenopausal and are undergoing chemotherapy and/or hormonal therapy for control of their disease. It is thought to be caused by a decline in estrogen and other hormones. These symptoms can include hot flashes, night sweats, vaginal dryness, pain during intercourse, difficulty with bladder control, insomnia, and depression. Some patients use **complementary therapies** such as vitamins, soy products, or black cohosh to try to reduce symptoms. Currently, there aren't studies to give us definitive answers about the use of these supplements. It is worth talking to your doctor about his thoughts if you wish to consider taking any. Some patients find that taking a medication like venlafaxine (Effexor) can be helpful in reducing hot flashes. Wearing cotton clothing in layers that can be peeled off as needed also can be a useful measure on your part. There are various vaginal lubricants that can be used for vaginal dryness and pain during intercourse. These include Replens, Astroglide, or K-Y Jelly. Avoid using petroleum-based products as they can increase risk of vaginal infections. Avoid spicy foods, smoking, alcohol, caffeine, hot showers, and hot weather, all of which can trigger hot flashes.

Complementary therapy

Interventions used in conjunction with standard therapies.

63. My dentures aren't fitting right and have caused ulcers on my gums. What caused this?

Mucositis

A condition in which the mucosa (the lining of the digestive tract, from the mouth to the anus) becomes swollen, red, and sore. For example, sores in the mouth that can be a side effect of chemotherapy.

This is known as **mucositis**, or mouth sores. It is an inflammation of the inside of the mouth and throat and can result in painful ulcers. Medications like steroids may increase the risk of developing an infection in your mouth. Keep your mouth clean and moist to prevent infection. Brush your teeth with a soft-bristled toothbrush after each meal and rinse regularly. Avoid commercial mouthwashes that contain alcohol because they can irritate the mouth. If you wear dentures that are not fitting properly, you will be more likely to get sores in your mouth from rubbing and irritation. This can be a particular problem if you have experienced or are experiencing weight loss because your gums may shrink changing the fit of your dentures. See your dentist for evaluation of this. If you have dental needs that have not been taken care of prior to starting chemotherapy, ask your oncologist and dentist to talk on the phone and discuss what strategy to use to reduce risk of infection and mouth sores while receiving your treatments.

64. I'm taking so many different medications now that my stomach is always upset. What can I do to feel better and be able to eat and enjoy food again?

Antiemetics

Drugs to stop or prevent nausea or vomiting.

Nausea and vomiting are relatively common side effects associated with chemotherapy drugs. With the development of anti-nausea medicines (called **antiemetics**), the incidence of nausea and vomiting has reduced considerably. When beginning new medications, such as hormonal therapy, these side effects may be problematic for a while. Pain medications have a reputation for contributing to nausea, too. Severe nausea that interferes with your ability to eat or retain foods can cause dehydration. Changes in what you eat and drink may be useful in managing nausea and vomiting.

Some specific suggestions include:

Eat a light meal before each chemotherapy treatment.

Have small amounts of food and liquids at a time.

Have bland foods and liquids.

Eat dry crackers when feeling nauseated.

Limit the amount of liquids you take with your meals.

Maintain adequate liquids in between meals; take mostly clear liquids such as water, apple juice, herbal tea, or bouillon.

Eat cool foods or foods at room temperature.

Avoid foods with strong odors.

Avoid high fat, greasy, and fried foods.

Avoid spicy foods, alcohol, and caffeine.

Suck on peppermint candies to help reduce or prevent nausea.

Rub peppermint flavored lip balm above your lips and below your nose so that you are smelling mint, which may reduce nausea.

Ask your oncologist for a prescription for an antiemetic and ask if you can take it in a preventative manner to prevent, reduce, and control nausea. These medicines include such drugs as Zofran, Kytril, and Compazine.

Changes in what you eat and drink may be useful in managing nausea and vomiting.

65. My feet and hands have gotten tingly. What is this, and how can I make it go away?

Peripheral neuropathy

Numbness and pain of the hands and feet, which can be caused by infection, very strong drugs (such as chemotherapy), or disease.

Neurological problems, such as **peripheral neuropathy**, are possible side effects of some chemotherapy drugs. Peripheral neuropathy is damage to peripheral nerves. There are three types of peripheral nerves: sensory, motor, and autonomic. Sensory nerves allow us to feel temperature, pain, vibration, and touch. Motor nerves are responsible for voluntary movement and allow us to walk and open doors, for example. Autonomic nerves control involuntary or automatic functions such as breathing, digestion of food, and bowel and bladder activities. When there is damage to the peripheral nerves, the symptoms depend on the types of peripheral nerves affected. Though chemotherapy drugs can affect any of the peripheral nerves, the most common ones affected are the sensory nerves causing numbness and tingling in the hands and feet. For patients who already have peripheral neuropathy from other causes, diabetes, for example, the chemotherapy can sometimes make it worse.

Symptoms of peripheral neuropathy include:
Numbness and tingling, which may feel like pins and needles in your hands and/or feet
Burning pain in hands and feet
Difficulty writing or buttoning a shirt
Difficulty holding a cup or glass
Constipation
Decreased sensation of hot or cold
Muscle weakness
Decreased hearing or ringing in the ears (known as tinnitus)

If you develop any of these symptoms, it's important to tell your doctor right away. Describe the symptoms you are experiencing. If you already have any of these symptoms before starting chemotherapy, tell your doctor. Your doctor may decide to prescribe medication for you to reduce these symptoms. The medicines most commonly used are drugs that are given to neurology patients for treatment of seizures and depression. Some examples are gabapentin (Neurontin), carbamazepine (Tegretol), and amitriptyline (Elavil). Additional measures you should consider taking at home include paying close attention when you walk and avoid having scatter rugs in your house. Keep your home well-lit so you can see where you are walking. If you are still driving a car, be sure you can feel the foot pedals. If temperatures are hard to decipher, then ask for help in checking the temperature of the bathwater as well as any hot beverages you are drinking. Take extra precaution to guard against frostbite in the water.

66. I am feeling more joint pain and backaches that make it difficult to walk around. What can I do to manage my pain?

For some patients, pain may be the most difficult symptom to overcome and cope with. Metastatic breast cancer that has spread to the bones, for example, can cause bone pain that is very uncomfortable. It can reach a point of making it difficult to walk around and function well because the pain is so intense. A primary goal for you and your doctor is to prevent pain from being debilitating if it happens. Your doctor will prescribe pain medications for you. Sometimes it takes several different types of medications to get pain under control. This is usually more of an issue for patients toward the end of life. If taking narcotics for pain management, avoid driving as your alertness may be impaired and you may be more prone to accidents. Some pain medications can be constipating so talk with your doctor about taking stool softeners to prevent bowel problems. The goal is for pain to be manageable and not so uncomfortable that your quality of life is negatively affected. Tell your doctor if the pain medications are no longer working as well as they did when first prescribed. Adjusting medications is a continuous and expected process.

67. I am so worried about pain. Will I suffer a lot?

Not everyone with metastatic cancer has pain. However, if you do have pain, rest assured that your doctor will be able to control it. The cancer itself does not cause pain. People with metastatic cancer experience pain if the tumor presses on surrounding organs or nerves. One of the major goals of systemic anti-cancer treatment is to control pain, but it may take a couple of months for it to be effective. While you are waiting for this, you will need specific anti-pain treatment. Sometimes the treatment does not kill enough cancer cells to make the pain go away completely, and you will have to continue to take pain medication.

Doctors use medicines and radiation therapy to control pain. The medicines are usually given by mouth, but they are sometimes administered in the veins or by placing medicated patches on the skin. Nerve blocks are often useful in controlling pain that is in a localized area. Relaxation techniques, massage, and acupuncture also have roles in managing some types of cancer pain.

68. How will my doctor control my bone pain?

Bone metastases are the most common cause of pain in patients with metastatic breast cancer. Not everyone with cancer in the bones has pain. Radiation therapy is particularly effective in treating bone pain. You may not experience its full effect until a few weeks after the last treatment, so be patient. In the meantime, you should not hesitate to take the pain medicine (**analgesics**) that your doctor prescribes. If you need narcotic medications to control your pain, your doctor may also want you to take an **NSAID (nonsteroidal anti-inflammatory drug)** to make it work better. Of course, the best way to ultimately control and prevent bone pain is for your cancer to go into remission from systemic therapy. Since radiation can make the side effects of chemotherapy worse (especially bone marrow suppression, mucositis, and diarrhea), your oncologist often holds off giving you chemotherapy during the radiation treatments. Your doctor may also recommend radiation therapy to prevent you from breaking a bone, even if the cancer in your bones is not causing pain. Intravenous bisphosphonates, such as pamidronate (Aredia) or zoledronic acid (Zometa), also help control bone pain and speed bone healing.

Analgesic
Drugs that reduce pain.

Nonsteroidal anti-inflammatory drugs (NSAIDs)
A class of pain medications, often sold over-the-counter, that includes ibuprofen and similar common painkillers.

69. Is it true that the bisphosphonates that I take for my bones will damage my jaw?

Osteonecrosis of the jaw is a painful disorder caused by loss of blood to the bone tissue, and eventual collapse of the jawbone. Recent reports have linked it to the use of intravenous bisphosphonates, but it appears to occur in very few breast cancer patients who are given

Osteonecrosis
When some noncancerous bone cells die off in a way that is not normal.

intravenous bisphosphonates for their bone metastases. The risk is increased in patients who have received prolonged doses of intravenous bisphosphonates, especially in conjunction with chemotherapy and corticosteroids. Additional risk factors include a history of jaw trauma, dental surgery, periodontal (gum) disease, or dental infections. For that reason, doctors recommend that you have a good dental exam with preventive dentistry intervention before you start intravenous bisphosphonate therapy. You should also try to avoid dental procedures during your treatment.

Most oncologists feel that the benefits of intravenous bisphosphonate treatments far outweigh the minimal risk of jaw osteonecrosis. Though it does not effect overall survival, intravenous bisphosphonate infusions significantly decrease skeletal events (fractures, pain) in breast cancer patients who have bone metastases. Either pamidronate (Aredia) or zoledronic acid (Zometa) is effective, but zoledronic acid is probably slightly better. In addition, it can be infused over 15 minutes and is, therefore, more convenient to get than pamidronate, which has to be given over 2 to 3 hours. Both drugs are given in the outpatient setting every 3–5 weeks.

Your doctor may want you to take calcium and vitamin D while you are getting these treatments. She will also measure your blood calcium, phosphorous, and magnesium levels at periodic intervals to make sure that they are normal. The bisphosphonates can adversely affect your kidneys, especially zoledronic acid, and your doctor will need to monitor your kidney function with blood tests. Both zoledronic acid and pamidronate are also used to lower the amount of calcium in patients with too much calcium in the blood (hypercalcemia) caused by metastatic breast cancer.

70. How will my doctor treat the swelling and pain that I have in my abdomen?

If your cancer spreads to the lining of your abdomen (peritoneum) you may develop ascites. Just like a child's bruised knee weeps fluid, tumor implants irritate the peritoneum and cause it to weep. The fluid that collects in the abdominal cavity is called **ascites**. It may cause swelling, pressure, and pain. The best way to control ascites is with systemic anti-cancer therapy, but your doctor may also use diuretics (water pills) and pain pills. Occasionally, your doctor may put a needle into your abdomen (paracentesis) to remove some fluid, but this is only a temporary solution since the fluid usually comes back within days to weeks.

Ascites
A build up of fluid in the abdominal cavity.

71. My husband and I have enjoyed an active sex life. Since my treatments have gotten more intense, this has been more difficult. What can we do to be able to still be sexually intimate? We both miss it.

The percentage of women dealing with metastatic breast cancer who are experiencing problems continuing sexual activity isn't clearly known. Even for the general population of women not dealing with anything as serious as metastatic breast cancer, 43 percent have reported problems with sexual activity. Some patients find it very difficult to comfortably discuss this issue with their doctor, though it may be very important to their quality of life. Side effects from treatment may result in lowering your libido or because of hair loss, weight gain, fatigue, or other symptoms, you simply don't feel well enough to try or confident enough with your self-esteem to engage in sexual activity. Physical intimacy is one aspect of a loving relationship. It gives us personal pleasure and creates a feeling of closeness to our partner. Sexual intercourse is just one way of being physically intimate. Cuddling, hugging, touching, rubbing, and holding hands are all pleasurable ways of showing one another affection. Talk with your partner about your concerns and feelings. This will help both of you to know how to help each other. Experiment with different positions. You may find one to be more comfortable than another when having sex. Vaginal lubricants (refer to page 71 regarding menopausal symptoms) can help with vaginal dryness. Some women who have not had success with vaginal lubricants have tried egg whites for lubrication. Be sure to wash thoroughly after intercourse but do not use douche solutions. If lack of energy impairs sexual activity, plan ahead for intimacy by identifying when you are feeling higher levels of energy during certain times of the day or week. Vaginal discharge, burning, or itching may be signs of a vaginal infection. See your gynecologist if you develop these symptoms so they can be properly treated.

Sexual intercourse is just one way of being physically intimate. Cuddling, hugging, touching, rubbing, and holding hands are all pleasurable ways of showing one another affection.

PART SEVEN

Targeted Therapy

What is a monoclonal antibody?

What is biologic targeted therapy,
and how does it work?

More . . .

72. What is a monoclonal antibody?

Antibodies

Special proteins produced by your immune system. They help protect the body from disease.

Antibodies are a type of protein. The immune system produces them in response to foreign substances that may be a threat to the body, for example, chemicals, virus particles, bacterial toxins, or cancer. These foreign substances are called **antigens**. Each type of antibody is unique and defends the body against one specific type of antigen. Because an antibody binds only to a specific antigen, it can act as a homing device to a tumor cell. The term monoclonal means from one specific type of cell. Monoclonal antibodies may be able to kill tumor cells themselves, or they may be linked with tumor killing substances. That "piggyback" system may allow treatment substances, such as drugs or radioactive materials, to be delivered directly to the tumor. Trastuzumab (Herceptin) therapy for HER2-positive breast cancer is one example of targeted therapy with monoclonal antibodies to treat metastatic breast cancer.

73. What is HER2-positive breast cancer, and how do I know if I have it?

Each normal breast cell contains the HER2 gene, which helps normal cells grow. The HER2 (also called HER2/neu or cERB-b2) gene is found in the DNA of a cell. This gene contains the information for making the HER2 protein receptor on the cell's surface. In normal cells, the HER2 protein receptor helps send growth signals from outside the cell to the inside of the cell. These signals tell the cell to grow and divide. Some breast cancer cells have an abnormally high number of HER2 genes per cell. When this happens, too much HER2 protein appears on the surface of these cancer cells. This overexpression of the HER2 protein causes cancer cells to grow and divide more quickly.

HER2-positive cancers are those that overexpress the HER2 protein receptor. Approximately 25 percent of breast cancer patients have HER2-positive tumors. It is very important for you and your doctor to know if your breast cancer is one of these. If it is, your treatment program will most likely contain trastuzumab (Herceptin), a monoclonal antibody that blocks the effects of the growth factor receptor protein HER2.

Your cancer's HER2 status is determined by analyzing your breast cancer tissue in the laboratory. Pathologists will run tests either on the primary breast cancer tissue removed at the time of your breast surgery, or on material obtained from a biopsy of one of your metastases. There are two methods of testing for HER2 tumor status; **immunohistochemistry (IHC)** and **fluorescence in situ hybridization (FISH)**. The scoring for an IHC test is from 0 to 3+. Zero and 1+ are HER2 negative; 2+ is a borderline or equivocal result; and 3+ is HER2 positive. FISH is a gene-based test used to determine the number of HER2 genes in the cells of the tumor. Though it is not a perfect test, it is generally regarded as the definitive test for HER2 overexpression. It is usually only done when the IHC result is borderline (2+).

74. What is biologic targeted therapy, and how does it work?

In recent years, scientists have made great strides in understanding the complicated biological pathways that cause cancer to develop, grow, and spread. They use drugs that block specific biological pathways and proteins involved in the growth and spread of cancer. Because they are "smart drugs" that focus on molecular and cellular changes that are specific to cancer, targeted cancer therapies may be more

Immunohisto-chemistry (IHC)

The most commonly used test to see if a tumor has too much of the HER2 receptor protein on the surface of the cancer cells. The IHC test gives a score of 0 to 3+ that indicates the amount of HER2 receptor protein. It also measures the presence of hormone receptors on the breast cancer cell too and determines if a tumor is hormone receptor positive or negative.

Fluorescence in situ hybridization (FISH)

This is a lab test that measures the amount of a certain gene in cells. It can be used to see if an invasive cancer has too many HER2 genes. A cancer with too many of these genes is called HER2-positive.

effective than traditional chemotherapy and less harmful to normal cells. Those used to treat metastatic breast cancer include trastuzumab (Herceptin) and lapatinib (Tykerb).

Drugs that target the hormone (estrogen and progesterone) receptors found on many breast cancer cells are among the oldest forms of breast cancer treatment.

Drugs that target the hormone (estrogen and progesterone) receptors found on many breast cancer cells are among the oldest forms of breast cancer treatment. This type of breast cancer uses female hormones to fuel its growth. Drugs like tamoxifen and fulvestrant block the estrogen receptor so that the cancer cells cannot get enough fuel and the cancer cells die. Other anti-estrogens, like the aromatase inhibitors anastrozole, decrease the amount of estrogen in postmenopausal women by blocking the aromatase enzyme needed to make estrogen. These work differently than the biologic targeted therapies do however.

Many of the biologic targeted therapy drugs block specific enzymes or growth factor receptors (GFRs) found on many cancer cells. The monoclonal antibody trastuzumab (Herceptin) does this by blocking the effects of the growth factor receptor protein HER2. Because the HER2 protein transmits growth signals to breast cancer cells, trastuzumab is an active drug in the 25 percent of breast cancer patients who have too much HER2. In metastatic breast cancer, trastuzumab can be given as a single agent, but it is usually used initially with traditional chemotherapy drugs like paclitaxel.

Lapatinib (Tykerb) is a small molecule that inhibits HER2 proteins. Because it has a different mechanism of action than trastuzumab, lapatinib is useful in patients with HER2-positive breast cancer whose breast cancer has progressed following treatment on anthracycline, taxane, and trastuzumab. Unlike trastuzumab, it is an oral drug. It is usually given in combination with capecitabine.

PART EIGHT

Clinical Trials

What is a "Clinical Trial," and am I a candidate to still participate in one if I have metastatic breast cancer?

What questions should I ask the doctor about a specific clinical trial he has recommended for me?

How do I find out about clinical trials that might be appropriate for me to consider?

More . . .

75. What is a "Clinical Trial," and am I a candidate to participate in one if I have metastatic breast cancer?

There are many different kinds of clinical trials. They range from studies focusing on ways to prevent, detect, diagnose, treat, and control breast cancer to studies that address quality of life issues.

There are many different kinds of clinical trials. They range from studies focusing on ways to prevent, detect, diagnose, treat, and control breast cancer to studies that address quality of life issues. Most clinical trials are carried out in phases. Each phase is designed to learn different information and build on the information previously discovered. Patients may be eligible for studies in different phases depending on their stage of disease (including stage IV breast cancer), therapies anticipated, as well as treatment they have already had. Patients are monitored at specific intervals while participating in studies.

Jessica's comments:

Participating in a clinical trial was important for me because I realize that by doing so not only am I potentially benefiting myself but also may be helping to establish the new treatment options for women who come after me.

76. What are the various study phases of clinical trials?

Phase I studies are used to find how much of a new drug can be given safely. In such studies only a small number of patients are asked to participate. When other treatments are no longer working to control your metastatic breast cancer, you may become a candidate to participate in such a trial. They are offered to patients whose cancer cannot be helped by other known treatment modalities. Some patients have received benefits from participation but most have experienced no benefits in fighting their cancer. Those who participate in phase I studies are paving the way for the next generation, which is important. Once the optimum dose is chosen, the drug is studied for its ability to shrink tumors in phase II trials.

Phase II studies are designed to find out if the treatment actually kills cancer cells in patients. A slightly larger group of patients is selected for this trial, usually between 20 and 50. Patients whose breast cancer has no longer responded to other known treatments may be offered participation in this type of trial. Tumor shrinkage is measured and patients are closely observed to measure the effects the treatment is having on her disease. Some patients may benefit from participation in phase II studies and others may not.

Phase III studies usually compare standard treatments already in use with treatments that appeared to be effective in phase II trials. This phase requires large numbers of patients to participate, usually thousands. Patients are normally **randomized** for the treatment regimen they will be receiving. These studies are seeking the benefits of longer survival, better quality of life, fewer side effects, and fewer cases of cancer recurrence.

Randomized
Describes the process in a clinical trial in which animal or human subjects are assigned by chance to separate groups that allow for comparison of different treatments.

Supportive care studies are tailored to improve ways of managing side effects caused by treatment. They also include some quality of life studies as well.

You may be a candidate for clinical trials in any of these categories so ask your doctor about clinical trials and see what studies you may qualify to participate in. Over time you may actually participate in several.

You may derive substantial benefit from participating in clinical trials. Every successful cancer treatment being used today started as a clinical trial. The patients who participated in these studies were the first to benefit. Hopefully, you will be in the next group of patients to benefit from clinical trials that are presented to you for consideration.

77. What questions should I ask the doctor about a specific clinical trial she has recommended for me?

Ask your doctor the following questions:

What is the purpose of the study?

How many people will be included in the study?

What does the study involve? What kinds of tests and treatment will I have?

How are treatments given, and what side effects might I expect?

What are the risks and benefits of each protocol?

What are the alternatives to the study?

How long will the study last?

What type of long term follow-up care is provided for those who participate?

Will I incur any costs? Will my insurance company pay for part of this?

When will the results be known?

How will you determine if this study is specifically benefiting me, if that is the goal?

If I'm not alive to hear the final results of the study, how can my family learn about the results of the study if they are interested?

This last question is a tough one to ask, because obviously the hope is that the drugs they are using will enable you to live in harmony with your breast cancer and survive a long time. There are some studies that are intended for participation after the patient has passed away. An example of such a study is the "Rapid Autopsy Program." It may be hard to imagine having such a clinical trial discussed with you but it is a very significant study that hopes to provide answers as to how breast cancer spreads from the breast to other organs and how it goes about sometimes changing its physiological features, such as changing from being hormone receptor positive to hormone receptor negative. Women participating in this trial agree to have tissue harvested from the organs upon their death, where it is known that the cancer has migrated. This enables researchers to study the tissue and learn the process whereby breast cancer travels and changes its behavior. This can result in learning and developing better treatments for women with metastatic disease. The ultimate goal is to be able to prevent the breast cancer from being able to ever leave the breast in the first place. If this can one day be achieved, then virtually no one would develop metastatic breast cancer and, in turn, no one would die of it. Such a trial obviously doesn't benefit the patient herself but can make a huge difference for the next generation of women who come after her.

The ultimate goal is to be able to prevent the breast cancer from being able to ever leave the breast in the first place.

78. How do I find out about clinical trials that might be appropriate for me to consider?

You can get information from your doctor but you can also do some homework yourself. Visit the following websites for more information:

1. National Comprehensive Cancer Network (NCCN) at *www.nccn.org*. You can also use this website to find a cancer center in your geographic region. Contact the center to see if there are any available clinical trials for individuals with metastatic

breast cancer. Some trials may be specific for women with stable disease and others may be for patients who have disease progression.

2. National Cancer Institute at *www.cancer.gov/ clinicaltrials/* or call 800-4-CANCER.

3. National Institutes of Health at *www.clinicaltrials .gov.* Select "focused search" button and type in "metastatic breast cancer."

4. Coalition of National Cancer Cooperative Groups at *www.cancertrialshelp.org* or call 877-520-4457.

5. Centerwatch also provides a list of clinical trials at *www.centerwatch.com.*

PART NINE

Complementary and Alternative Medicine

What are examples of some complementary and alternative treatments that I might hear about or want to learn more about?

I want to try some complementary therapies while receiving my chemo treatments. How do I go about deciding which therapies to do?

Where can I go to get credible information that is up-to-date related to research studies that have been done regarding complementary and alternative medicine?

More . . .

79. *What are complementary and alternative treatments?*

Complementary and alternative medicine (CAM) is also sometimes referred to as integrative medicine and covers a wide variety of approaches and techniques with the goal of improving health and treating disease. These treatments are not recognized as standard of care or part of conventional treatment by the traditional medical community. When such treatments and methods are used with conventional treatment they are usually referred to as complementary; when used instead of traditional treatment they are considered to be alternative.

80. *I've heard that some alternative medicine treatments may actually cure cancer. Is this true?*

It can be difficult sometimes to conduct evidence-based medicine clinical trials on these methods of treatment because there may not be clear-cut measurements that can tell us how effective they are in an isolated manner. For example, someone may be doing some form of complementary medicine while also getting other standard treatment. How do you determine which did what? More and more scientifically based research is being done now and some therapies have been proven to be beneficial for cancer patients. There are lots of websites that claim something works. They may be self reporting by a company and not credible conducted studies that are evidence-based and conducted in the rigid manner in which clinical trials are to be carried out. These claims sound wonderful and even imply that it's a "cure for breast cancer" when there may be nothing that scientifically supports those claims. Be cautious of

Complementary and alternative medicine (CAM)

Forms of treatment that are used in addition to, or instead of, standard treatments. Their purpose is to strengthen your whole mind and body to maximize your health, energy, and well-being. These practices are not considered "standard" medical approaches. They include dietary supplements, vitamins, herbal preparations, special teas, massage therapy, acupuncture, spiritual healing, visualization, and meditation.

advertisements that claim that for a fee they will mail you the cure for your cancer. If what they were selling really was a cure then an NCI-designated cancer center would be offering it and telling you about it. The U.S. government founded the National Center for Complementary and Alternative Medicine (NCCAM) as part of the National Institutes of Health with the intended goal of providing information about what is safe and effective regarding these types of therapies. Ask your doctors for their input regarding information you have read about or heard so you can weed out accurate information from claims that may not be correct. There are some types of therapies that would interfere with the treatments he has given you. For example, certain vitamins in high doses may impair the effect of some chemotherapy drugs. There are other types of therapies that your doctor may encourage you to do, such as **acupuncture** or yoga.

Most published breast cancer studies that you will find will have been done with women who have not developed metastatic disease. These studies may have looked at the potential benefit in preventing recurrence. Don't become frustrated by this. They still may be useful to consider and discuss with your doctor even if there aren't solid data to demonstrate if they may be specifically useful for you.

Ask your doctors for their input regarding information you have read about or heard so you can weed out accurate information from claims that may not be correct.

81. What are examples of some complementary and alternative treatments that I might hear about or want to learn more about?

Complementary and alternative medicines may be categorized in many different ways. The NCCAM divides these therapies and treatments into five categories:

Acupuncture

The technique of inserting thin needles into the skin at specific points. This can help control pain and other symptoms for some individuals and is a form of ancient Chinese medicine. It is a form of complementary therapy.

1. Alternative medical systems of theory and practice. Many of these are used by various Native American tribes. Acupuncture originated as a part of traditional Chinese medicine. Other examples of alternative medical systems are homeopathic and naturopathic medicine.

2. Mind-body interventions. These are techniques that aim at helping the mind to enhance various body functions and reduce symptoms. Examples include relaxation, **meditation**, guided imagery, hypnosis, prayer, and support groups.

3. Biological-based therapies. These include dietary (for example, macrobiotic diet), herbal (for example, palmetto), biologic (for example, shark cartilage), and orthomolecular (for example, vitamins) treatments.

4. Manipulative and body-based methods. These are techniques that involve manipulation or movement of the body, such as those used by chiropractors and massage therapists.

5. Energy therapies. These are techniques that manipulate energy fields within or outside of the body, such as therapeutic touch, Reiki, or magnets.

Meditation

A mental technique that clears the mind and relaxes the body through concentration.

The use of complementary and alternative therapies is rapidly increasing. This is partly due to our increasing desire to help ourselves and utilize more "natural" methods of treating and preventing disease. There is valuable, scientifically based information about some forms of CAM that confirm some are useful. It is also felt that an increased use of complementary and alternative therapies is a sign that may represent our personal feelings of desperation that many people feel when dealing with metastatic disease. It means we are perhaps willing to try anything and everything we feel may help us. Complementary and alternative therapies are not regulated in the same manner that medications and medical devices are. Some pills you see that claim to do certain things may not do anything or potentially may even be harmful to you.

82. I want to try some complementary therapies while receiving my chemo treatments. How do I go about deciding which therapies to do?

Discuss with your doctor your thoughts on this and inform him that you want to try some complementary therapies. Many, like yoga and prayer, can be done and are safe to use with traditional treatment. If you have read about a particular therapy that interests you, bring that information with you to your doctor for his review so that he understands your interest and what you are hoping to accomplish by engaging in this therapy. Therapies that may raise questions about safety and benefit are biologic treatments, in particular.

83. My disease is progressing and I'm running out of options for treatment. Can I embark on alternative medicine and do it on my own?

It is a patient's right to be able to do whichever treatments she desires, whether her oncologist agrees with her or not. There are some patients who take the alternative medicine road right from the start and refuse any form of standard traditional treatment for their metastatic breast cancer. Their clinical outcome is usually grave. Things may seem fine initially until the disease

It is a patient's right to be able to do whichever treatments she desires, whether her oncologist agrees with her or not.

begins to pick up more speed in spreading to other organ sites within the body. It is much harder to get control of breast cancer if it involves multiple organ sites and is growing fast. There may be a point, after traditional treatment has been exhausted and control of the disease is no longer possible, when patients will embark on other routes of treatment on their own. Your doctor should understand this, but he or she will also want you to have realistic expectations. The chance of it helping is small, and the objective is for it to not hinder you. The power of the mind should never be underestimated. If we believe we are benefiting from something then we may be. It will be relieving for everyone when more scientifically based research is completed and published to better guide us as to what is wise to do and what may not be in the future.

84. Where can I go to get credible, up-to-date information about research studies that have been done regarding complementary and alternative medicine?

It is important to have the latest information because this is an ever-changing area of study. The following websites provide good, reliable information:

1. Cancer Information Services of the National Cancer Institute at *www.cancer.gov/cancerinfo/treatment/cam*.

2. National Center for Complementary and Alternative Medicine of the National Institutes of Health at *www.nccam.nih.gov/health*.

3. Memorial Sloane–Kettering Cancer Center at *www.mskcc.org/aboutherbs*.

4. M. D. Anderson Cancer Center at *www.mdanderson.org/topics/complementary.*

5. American Academy of Medical Acupuncture at *www.medicalacupuncture.org* or 323-937-5514.

The following sources provide information specifically on dietary supplements, including vitamins, minerals, and botanicals:

1. Office of Dietary Supplements of the National Institutes of Health at *www.dietary-supplements.info.nih.gov.*

2. Center for Food Safety and Applied Nutrition of the US Food and Drug Administration (FDA) at *www.cfsan.fda.gov.*

3. American Botanical Council at *www.herbalgram.org.*

4. The National Library of Medicine at *www.nih.gov/nccam/camonpubmed.html* offers scientific bibliographic citations related to particular therapies.

85. How do I make the decision if I should or shouldn't use one of the complementary or alternative therapies my family and friends are recommending?

First, do your homework and learn more about the therapy before jumping in and trying it, particularly if it involves taking a product of some type. Some specific questions to think about are:

1. Do the promises sound too good to be true? Is here conflicting information about how beneficial this therapy is and its actual benefit?

2. What is the evidence supporting the claims of its effectiveness? Has a rigorous scientific evidence-based study been conducted and published in a credible cancer journal? Or is the information about its effectiveness only anecdotal, based on satisfied customers who have purchased the product?

3. What are the risks of using this treatment? How safe is it? How was safety evaluated for this product/therapy?

4. If someone is providing this therapy, what are his or her credentials to do so? Does he or she have a certification or a license? Some practitioners are licensed by state medical boards or accredited by professional organizations.

5. Is the source of the therapy also the seller of the therapy? If so, they may have a vested interest in convincing people to purchase it. Sadly, some dishonest people will prey on individuals who are dealing with end-stage cancers.

There are two websites that provide tips to help you make decisions about the use of complementary and alternative medicine.

1. National Center for Complementary and Alternative Medicine of the National Institutes of Health at *www.nccam.nih.gov/health/decisions/index.htm.*

2. Center for Food Safety and Applied Nutrition of the U.S. Food and Drug Administration at *www.cfan.fda.gov/~dms/ds-savvy.html.*

Before making any decisions to try something on your own, most specifically if it involves taking a product, discuss it with your doctor.

PART TEN

Other Common Questions

My family wants me to stop smoking, but I already have incurable cancer. Do I have to stop?

A friend of mine who has metastatic disease says that periodically she gets to stop treatment for a while. How does my oncologist decide if I can have a drug holiday? How long does it usually last?

Should I still get my annual screening mammogram?

More . . .

86. My family wants me to stop smoking, but I already have incurable cancer. Do I have to stop?

You are not going to make your cancer worse by continuing to smoke, but there is some controversy on whether or not cigarette smoking makes the side effects of treatment worse. This is probably true of radiation therapy that involves any part of the upper gastrointestinal tract, especially the mouth and esophagus. Smoking is a well-known risk factor for pulmonary complications following general anesthesia for surgery. It may also increase your risk of developing blood clots or pulmonary emboli while on hormonal therapy. Although some oncologists believe that it increases the severity of mucositis (mouth sores and ulcers) from chemotherapy, studies have shown that this effect is minimal, at most. Indeed, most studies have failed to show any dramatic increase in the side effects of most chemotherapy drugs in people who smoke, compared to those who do not.

Stopping smoking is hard enough to do under the best of circumstances, and these are hardly the best of circumstances. On the other hand, some people getting chemotherapy do lose the taste for cigarettes. Others find that their diagnosis is just the motivation that they need to stop, especially when they see it as a way of setting a good example for their loved ones and friends. After all, they have everything to gain by kicking the habit. Even if your family members do not smoke, your smoke can jeopardize their health (*passive smoking*). If you are able to stop smoking, you will probably feel better, and that does go a long way to helping you handle the stresses of chemotherapy and cancer. If your family wants you to stop, but you cannot, it probably is not worth the bad feelings that usually result from continuing to argue about it.

87. My doctor told me that I have a tumor in my liver. Is that the same as cancer?

Some doctors use words like "tumor," "spot," "neoplasm," or "mass" to ease the emotional blow of the word "cancer." However well meaning it may be, this type of paternalism is not helpful. You need to know in clear terms your cancer has returned so that you can make appropriate decisions about what to do to deal with this reality. If your doctor refuses to speak with you honestly and directly, you need to find another doctor who will.

On the other hand, doctors often use words like "mass" or "spot" to describe an abnormality on a scan that is suspicious for cancer, but could be something else. In situations like this, your doctor will suggest a biopsy to confirm his suspicions. After a pathologist looks at this biopsy, your doctor will be able to tell you if it is cancer or not.

If your doctor refuses to speak with you honestly and directly, you need to find another doctor who will.

88. I have liver cancer. Is it true that it is a death sentence?

It is important to understand that breast cancer that has spread (metastasized) to the liver is not the same as liver cancer; lung metastases are not lung cancer; brain metastases are not brain cancer; and bone metastases are not bone cancer. When cancer spreads (metastasizes) from one organ to another, it retains the characteristics of the place where it started out. A cancer that starts out in the liver (*primary* liver cancer) is completely different from a cancer that has spread (*secondary* or *metastatic* cancer) to the liver. Many cancers metastasize to the liver, but they all behave differently, depending upon where they started out. The treatment and chances of remission relate to the primary tumor site, not to where it has metastasized. Breast cancer is one of the most responsive cancers to

Prognosis

An estimation of the likely outcome of an illness based upon the patient's current status and the available treatments.

treatment and the **prognosis**, whether it is in the liver or bone or some other organ, is better than almost any other type of metastatic cancer. Breast cancer that has spread to the vital organs is usually more aggressive than breast cancer that has spread to the bone or soft tissues, but liver metastases are hardly an immediate "death sentence." Your chances of remissions are more related to how much treatment you have had in the past, how well it has worked, your general health, and the amount of metastatic disease that is in your body.

Your oncologist will help you choose the best overall treatment for your breast cancer. When breast cancer has metastasized to the liver, this usually involves chemotherapy or targeted therapy, but hormonal therapy may also be an option. Surgery or radiofrequency ablation (RFA) is sometimes used to treat localized liver metastases. RFA involves placing a needle probe, usually through the skin, directly into the liver metastasis and using heat to kill the cancer cells. Cryosurgery is a similar technique that kills the metastatic cells by freezing instead of heating. Another technique that is used less often is tumor chemoembolization, where chemotherapy is delivered directly to your liver metastases through a catheter that a radiologist passes into the liver by way of the artery in your groin.

89. A friend of mine who has metastatic disease says that periodically she gets to stop treatment for a while. How does my oncologist decide if I can have a drug holiday? How long does it usually last?

The standard practice of most oncologists is to continue chemotherapy for as long as it is working or until you have unacceptable side effects. However, you and your oncologist may decide to stop chemotherapy for a while, if you have metastatic disease that has been stable or in remission for some time. This may be particularly important to you if you are having considerable side effects from the chemotherapy.

There are not a lot of studies to help you make this decision, but the limited information available suggests that while continuous chemotherapy does not change **overall survival** it does prolong the time that your cancer stays in remission (**progression-free survival**) when compared to shorter course chemotherapy. The downside of this is that continuous chemotherapy is often associated with more side effects than shorter course chemotherapy. On the other hand, some people actually feel better getting chemotherapy.

Much of this depends upon the particular chemotherapy program that you are getting. For example, it is unusual for someone to get more than 6 months of paclitaxel without having significant numbness and tingling in her fingers or toes. This dose-related peripheral neuropathy could cause severe pain and interfere with your ability to hold objects or walk. In fact, one study showed little difference in the time to breast cancer progression in a group of patients who got long-term, compared to short-term, paclitaxel.

If your cancer recurs, but it is **asymptomatic** (for example, your re-staging bone scan shows a few new small spots in the bones, but you have no pain), it may be quite reasonable for you to take a chemotherapy holiday for a few months. Knowing that your cancer is progressing, you and your oncologist can closely monitor the situation with scans, blood tests, and routine visits so that you can begin a new treatment regimen at the first sign of symptoms or change in the cancer's rate of growth.

Overall survival

The percentage of people in a study who have survived for a certain period of time, usually reported as time since diagnosis or treatment. Often called the survival rate.

Progression-free survival

The length of time during and after treatment in which a patient is living with a disease that does not get worse. Progression-free survival may be used in a clinical study or trial to help find out how well a new treatment works.

Asymptomatic

Not manifesting any symptoms.

Emily's comments:

What a strange term—a drug holiday. But that is exactly what it is! I get to have a break for a while from taking medicines all the time. I feel that my body is getting a chance to recover from chemicals and I know that I'm being monitored closely to ensure that it is safe for me to take a break from treatment for a while.

90. Should I still get my annual screening mammogram?

If your doctor was at all concerned that your breast cancer metastases came from a new breast cancer in your other breast (second breast cancer primary), you probably had your last **mammogram** when your metastatic disease first appeared. If not, it was probably sometime within the preceding year. You will most likely never need to have another mammogram. The purpose of annual screening mammography is to find and cure early small breast cancers before they spread out of the breast. Now that you have metastatic breast cancer, that is no longer possible. Even if a mammogram found a second breast cancer primary, removing it would not affect the course of your present breast cancer metastases, their response to treatment, or your life expectancy. Your focus should now be on treating the life-threatening cancer that has spread from your breast.

Similarly, there is probably no reason for you to have routine colonoscopy to screen for colon cancer. In fact, this procedure can increase your risk of infection or bleeding complications from chemotherapy.

Mammogram

An X-ray examination of the breast.

The only problem that you might now have from a new breast cancer primary would be from skin breakdown, bleeding, or discomfort due to the local effects of a growing mass in the breast or under your arm. Even if a mammogram found a new small breast cancer today, it probably would not cause this type of problem for 3 to 5 years. It is most likely that you or your doctor would feel such a new breast cancer long before this occurred, and it is most likely that the treatment that you are getting for your breast cancer metastases is also treating any cancer cells that might be growing in the other breast.

PART ELEVEN

End of Life, Treatment, Crossroads, Making Plans

I don't know how to approach talking about such decisions with my family. How do I do this?

How and when will the doctor recommend that I stop treatment?

I feel very stressed about my medical situation and need time to clear my head and think about what I want to do. How can I do this?

More . . .

The goal of treatment of metastatic breast cancer is to sustain life while ensuring quality of life.

The goal of treatment of metastatic breast cancer is to sustain life while ensuring quality of life. There may be a point in time down the road when your doctor tells you news that you wish you didn't have to hear—that the treatments are no longer working and that there aren't any other treatments to offer. This is the toughest discussion you will ever experience and your doctor will ever have to do. It's shocking, depressing, overwhelming, frustrating, and not fair. But it happens. Some of the things that need to happen at this point in your journey are provided in this special chapter.

91. What is palliative care?

Palliative care is a philosophy of care that is intended to address your medical, physical, emotional, social, and spiritual needs. It is designed to help you have the best quality of life possible. Though originally created to be exclusively for patients at end of life, this type of approach to treatment and care is now available for patients in active treatment, too. A key component of this approach to care is helping to ensure that pain management is handled well. When pain is not able to be well controlled, the doctors may refer you to a palliative care specialist.

Advanced directives

Legal documents that allow people to express their decisions regarding what they do and don't want to have done during their last weeks or months in case they become unable to communicate effectively.

92. What is an advanced directive and how can I make sure my wishes are known?

Advanced directives are legal documents that allow you to state what type of medical care you want to receive if you become unable to make such decisions or speak on your own behalf in the future. Although the specific laws and terminology for advanced directives may vary from state to state, there are two basic types of advanced directives: A **living will** and a **healthcare proxy**.

93. What is a living will? Is it the same as a healthcare proxy?

No. A living will is a special document in which you give specific instructions regarding your healthcare, particularly focusing on measures that relate to prolonging your life. A living will can describe which medical interventions you want to have done as well as what you don't want performed based on specific circumstances. For example, if you were unable to eat or drink anymore, would you want to have artificial nutrition through a feeding tube or receive nourishment with an IV? If your heart were to stop would you want CPR performed? Would you want to be on a respirator?

It can be useful in making these types of decisions to differentiate between the types of medical problems that may occur. If the medical problems were treatable and reversible, you may want all measures taken to resuscitate you and support you. If the problem was one of progression of disease, and no treatments are available to help fight the cancer, you may not want to have extraordinary measures taken such as resuscitation to prolong your life. In that situation, some people want to be explicit about this and request to sign a "do not resuscitate" (DNR) order to ensure that none of these measures is taken. Making these types of decisions is very hard. Communicating them to your family members is important and an emotional challenge. It's important that your wishes are carried out, however, and this helps ensure that they are.

Living will

Outlines what care you want in the event you become unable to communicate due to coma or heavy sedation.

Healthcare proxy

Permits a designated person to make decisions regarding your medical treatment when you are unable to do so.

There are two limitations to a living will. Not all states recognize a living will. It is also impossible to imagine all the potential circumstances that might occur in the future regarding your health. There may be decisions that you simply haven't thought about yet or aren't ready to discuss and make decisions about. These types of problems may be alleviated by designating a healthcare proxy.

This is sometimes also referred to as a healthcare surrogate, a medical proxy, or a medical power of attorney. This person is authorized by you to make healthcare decisions on your behalf when you are not able to do so for yourself. He or she can decide which medical interventions will and won't be carried out, what will be performed, and what will be withheld. Though the terms vary from one state to another, all states recognize the term "healthcare proxy."

When choosing the person to serve in the important role as your healthcare proxy, be sure to choose someone you trust and who will make decisions based on what you want for yourself, not on what he or she wants for you or assume he or she would want in your situation. This person can be a family member or a friend. Talk with the person about what you want to have done in the event such decisions are needed. It's especially important to discuss issues regarding sustaining life with artificial means so your wishes are clearly known and understood. You can change your proxy at any time as well as change your decisions as you need and want.

Make your family and friends aware of whom you have chosen as your healthcare proxy. It's important for everyone to support this individual in making decisions on your behalf. If you have completed a living will (and this is wise for everyone to do, even unrelated to their medical condition), share this with them as well. Inform all of your doctors and other members of your medical team what your wishes are and give them copies of any advanced directive documents you have signed. Each time you become an inpatient, the staff should automatically ask you if you have such documents and if you brought them with you so they can become part of your medical record.

94. I don't know how to approach such decisions with my family. How do I do this?

Having a discussion about what you would want if you were unable to make decisions for yourself can be difficult for most people, but it is wise to do. Even women not dealing with metastatic breast cancer should be taking such steps since none of us knows when we may be in an auto accident or other medical crisis that warrants such decisions be made. You may want to discuss this with your loved ones but worry that it will upset them. You may worry that while discussing this important issue you will get upset. It is always better to discuss these things when you are feeling relatively well rather than waiting for a crisis to hit and having to discuss it at that time. This way you can calmly think about it, express your wants and needs, and be clear in what you want to happen.

It is always better to discuss these things when you are feeling relatively well rather than waiting for a crisis to hit and have to discuss it at that time.

There are various ways you might begin this discussion. You might say something like "I want to be sure that if I were ever to become more ill than I am now you would know what I want to have done." Sometimes family members don't agree with our decisions. This can make the discussion harder and, frankly, even more important to be clear and have things documented. This is a good reason for an advanced directive. Loved ones never want to picture you in a situation that warrants having to make decisions without you being able to speak for yourself.

95. How do I get the correct forms to complete an advanced directive?

You can obtain state-specific advanced directive forms from a lawyer, your doctor, or your local hospital. If you were to be admitted to the hospital and didn't have one already prepared, you would be offered one to complete and sign, which will apply to your care during that specific hospital admission.

The Partnership for Caring, a nonprofit organization whose mission is to improve how people die, also provides state-specific documents. They also provide information on end-of-life issues and offer a national crisis and information hotline regarding such issues. To reach them for more information call 800-989-9455 or check their website at *www.partnershipforcaring.org/Advance/index.html*.

96. How and when will the doctor recommend that I stop treatment?

There may be a time when you and your oncologist have a serious discussion about how your treatment has been going. It may include a discussion about treatments that are no longer working and the lack of additional treatment options available. You may want to stay on a particular drug regimen, but your doctor may have determined that the treatment is no longer effective.

The doctor may tell you that the benefits from taking the treatment are too small in comparison to the side effects you are experiencing and will continue to experience, thus affecting the quality of your remaining life in a major way. The two of you may decide to change pathways from aggressively fighting the disease to beginning to prepare for end of life. There is probably no harder decision than this to make. In some cases the patient makes the decision to end treatment herself. She may decide this based on how she feels and would rather focus on closure with family and friends and enjoy quality time with loved ones rather than continuing aggressive therapy.

There have been situations where no such discussion between the treating medical oncologist and the patient happens. This is truly unfortunate because treating for the sake of giving some type of treatment isn't factoring in the patient's personal goals and quality life needs. It's important to weigh the goals of treatment against the goals the patient has. Some patients expect the doctor to bring up the issue of stopping treatment and some doctors delay the discussion anticipating the patient will initiative the discussion. The result is that the patient doesn't always have the opportunity to prepare for end of life as she had anticipated, leaving family members to make decisions that they are not prepared to do. There are no rules about this and no specific guidelines to be followed. Some people decide to continue treatment until the last possible moment and others choose to stop earlier. Remember, the decision to stop treatment can be reversed if you wish. Talking with your family and doctors about it can help you decide what is realistic. It is appropriate to be optimistic about getting this disease under control. That is the goal, after all. If there is a time that realism takes over optimism, then making the decision can be done with you in a thoughtful way with your oncologist's help and family's support.

97. My doctor says that it's time to get hospice involved and stop my treatment. What is hospice and what can I expect them to help me with?

Hospice

An organization that provides programs and services designed to help alleviate the physical and psychosocial suffering associated with progressive, incurable illness.

Hospice tries to help the patient and her close family members prepare for end of life. Hospice's mission is to improve the quality of life for individuals with health problems that are considered fatal. Hospice helps with: 1) pain relief and other medical supportive care; 2) emotional and spiritual support for you and your family; and 3) help with daily tasks such as bathing, dressing, and other activities of daily living. They can also be instrumental in helping reduce financial expenses associated with end of life cancer care by obtaining prescription medicines at cost; arranging for a hospital bed, commode, wheelchair, and other medical equipment that may be needed at home; as well as provide hospice nurses and home health aides to come to you on a routine basis. For patients who prefer to not be in the home and would rather be in a hospice facility, your doctor will arrange for admission to such a place that will be as close to your home as possible, to make it convenient for your family and friends to see and spend time with you. Hospice facilities have an open door policy of permitting visitors 24/7. Hospice also provides spiritual counselors, depending on your religious faith and personal desires and needs. Many insurance companies cover hospice care. If you are over 65, you probably qualify for the Medicare hospice benefit. You may want to check with your insurance company if they have a relationship with specific hospice care units in your geographic region. For more information on hospice, call the Hospice Foundation of America at 800-854-3402.

Hospice's mission is to improve the quality of life for individuals with health problems that they are no longer able to treat and are considered fatal.

Tia's comments:

I worry about how my kids will cope with my dying. Though I admit I'm scared, I know it scares them even more. It's time I met with my hospice chaplain to discuss this and get some insight as to what they may be thinking and how I can get closure as well as feel that they will be okay after I'm gone. It's been wonderful how comfortable I have felt talking with the hospice staff. They are obviously much more experienced than I am in these things and I appreciate having them here for support and as a sounding board.

98. I want my children to remember me. I also want to help them cope with my having to leave them. What can you suggest to help us with both?

For children who are young, it's important for them to understand that nothing they have done has caused this to happen. Young children sometimes think they have wished this on their mother. They may have thought something like, "Mommy wouldn't let me play at Joey's house. I wish she were dead. She is mean to me." They think that they have literally managed to make this happen. Make it clear that nothing they have done has caused the cancer. Let them know that cancer is not contagious. Teens and pre-teens can feel a real sense of anxiety and distress. Older children who are out on their own, perhaps with their own families, will surely feel pain and loss but are better equipped emotionally to deal with this than young people are. For any children still living at home and dependent on you, emphasize to them that they will be taken care of, no matter what happens.

For children under the age of 21, consider getting cards for each of them—cards for each birthday up through age 21, graduation from high school, from college, cards for significant holidays you celebrate together, such as Easter, Christmas, Rosh Hashanah, cards for when they marry, and when they have their own first child. Write one sentence in each card that is specific for that date. What do you want to tell your child on this day (for example, when she turns sweet sixteen)? You can still be "right there" instilling your values in your children by doing this, and they will greatly value these cards as they grow up. In order to do this, you will need to recruit the assistance of the card store manager because some cards are seasonal (and stored in the back room). Explain your situation or, if you are not able to go yourself, ask a family member to go on your behalf. Put the name of the child and the date it is to be opened on the outside of the envelope and have them stored in a safety deposit box, rather than stored in your home. These are not replaceable later. If there were to be a flood or fire, they would be lost. It's worth the money each year to rent a safety deposit box at a local bank. Select a family member to be responsible for their timely distribution. Your children will sense your presence at the time of each milestone in their lives.

An additional idea for daughters is to create a charm bracelet for her that contains milestones she has already reached or favorite places the two of you have enjoyed together. Then purchase additional charms to be added later. A graduation cap for graduation from high school, a Sweet 16 charm for her 16th birthday, or wedding bells for when she marries.

Be sure your wishes are known regarding who you want to receive special mementos you own, such as specific pieces of jewelry. Don't leave this for your family to decipher alone, if it can be avoided. What you want done with these things is important for them to know. Your heart will tell you what to do. They certainly know it is not your choice to succumb to this disease. Fate has dealt you a hand that wasn't your doing or theirs. The verse below provides comfort to many family members, as well as to friends and even to patients who have metastatic breast cancer.

> *I stand at the shore—a ship spread her white sails to the morning breeze and starts for the blue ocean. She is an object of beauty and strength as I watch her like a speck of white cloud just where the sea and sky come down to mingle with each other. Then someone at my side says, "There, she is gone!"*
>
> *Gone? Gone where? Gone from my sight, that is all. She is just as large in mast and hull and spar as she was when she left my side...and just as able to bear her load of living freight to the place of her destination.*
>
> *Her diminished size is in me, not in her; and just at the moment that someone at my side says, "There, she is gone," there are other eyes watching and other voices ready to take up the glad shout, "Here she comes!"*
>
> —Henry Van Dyke

Lauren's comments:

Selecting cards for my children to have as they grow up without me was very hard at first. Then as I began to write in each one what my wishes were for them on that significant day in their lives, I felt better. This will be one of the ways I feel I will still be here for my children, instilling my value system in them, and telling them my hopes and dreams for their futures.

99. I feel very stressed about my medical situation and need time to clear my head and think about what I want to do. How can I do this?

Sometimes it is advisable to request to meet with a social worker or counselor for assistance. If you are involved with hospice, let the hospice staff taking care of you know you are distressed. This is not the time to hide it or try to see if the feelings of anxiety will pass. You are in an extraordinary situation and it is perfectly normal to feel upset. You need to find ways to relieve your stress and reduce your fears. Some ways to do this are:

1. Take a walk or exercise. Nothing strenuous, but power walking or treadmill walking are good options.

2. Keep a journal of your thoughts and feelings. Writing them down is very therapeutic.

3. Meditation, prayer, or performing relaxation exercises that include deep breathing is helpful.

4. Talk with someone such as a close friend, clergy, or counselor, about your fears and anxieties.

5. Consider joining a support group. Some breast centers offer special support groups for women dealing with metastatic disease.

6. Join an online support group.

7. Listen to soothing music or a CD of sounds like the ocean or birds chirping.

8. Create a work of art that displays your feelings and thoughts. There are some breast centers that offer art therapy. You don't have to be an artist to do this. A simple drawing or creation from clay can be done. It's your work of art. You don't have to share it with anyone unless you choose to do so.

9. Do yoga.

10. Spend time with close friends who you can be yourself with. Talk, read from a joke book, watch a funny movie, listen to music together, eat dessert. All of this is good for you, good for them, and good for the soul.

100. How do I decide what is the best way to be spending my time if the doctor tells me that my time is limited? Do I still work as much as I can? Do I take a trip? How do I make these decisions?

Often, as we are going through our daily routine, we don't realize how precious time is. It's not until we learn that we have a limited amount of it, that we recognize just how precious it is. Sit and talk with your loved ones about these decisions. You have the right to spend it as you want and not to feel pressure to maintain your old routine, especially if you were overloaded with responsibilities. If you enjoy doing these things, then do them. If you don't then, discuss with your family how you would prefer to spend your time. It may be seeing grandchildren more often. You may wish to take a trip. If that isn't realistic, based on how you are feeling, then get a movie (IMAX, if available) of the place you long to see and take a virtual trip there. This is a time to express your thoughts and feelings more openly and let people know what your concerns, wishes, and hopes are, especially for those who you will leave behind. For many this may be a spiritual time. For others it may be a time to spend resting with briefer visits by family and friends.

Table 1 Drugs Used in the Treatment of Breast Cancer

Drug Name Generic (Brand), Maker	Actions/Common Side Effects*
CHEMOTHERAPY	The treatment of cancer using specific chemical agents or drugs that are selectively destructive to malignant cells and tissues.
ALKYLATING AGENTS	Alkylating agents are a group of chemotherapy drugs that target the DNA of cancer cells to prevent the cells from growing or reproducing. Alkylating agents attack cancer cells in all phases and disrupt their growth. These cells are then destroyed.
Cyclophosphamide (Cytoxan) Bristol-Myers Squibb	Cyclophosphamide (Cytoxan) is a chemotherapy drug commonly used to treat breast cancer and other cancers. Cyclophosphamide first disrupts cancer cells, then destroys them. Cyclophosphamide is taken in tablets by mouth or intravenously (through the vein) over 30–60 minutes. Side effects may include decrease in blood cell counts with increased risk of infection; nausea, vomiting, diarrhea, and abdominal pain; decreased appetite; hair loss (reversible); bladder damage; fertility impairment; lung and hearing damage (with high doses); sores in mouth or on lips; and stopping of menstrual periods. Less common side effects: decreased platelet count (mild) with increased risk of bleeding, blood in urine, darkening of nail beds, acne, fatigue, fetal changes if patient becomes pregnant when taking cyclophosphamide. At high doses, can cause heart problems. Urinary system problems and some secondary cancers have been reported.
ANTHRACYCLINE ANTIBIOTICS	**Anthracyclines work by deforming the DNA structure of cancer cells and terminating their biological function. They disrupt the growth of cancer cells, which are then destroyed.**
Doxorubicin (Adriamycin) Pfizer	Doxorubicin (Adriamycin) is a type of antibiotic used specifically in the treatment of cancer. It interferes with the multiplication of cancer cells and slows or stops their growth and spread in the body. Side effects may include decreased white blood cell count with increased risk of infection, decreased platelet count with increased risk of bleeding, loss of appetite, darkening of nail beds and skin creases of hands, hair loss, damage to the skin if drug gets outside the veins, nausea, and vomiting. Less common side effects: sores in mouth or on lips, radiation recall skin changes, fetal abnormalities if taken while pregnant or if patient becomes pregnant while on this drug. Patients should be tested for heart problems before beginning doxorubicin and should be continuously monitored for developing problems during treatment.

*Drug information has been drawn from *The Physicians' Desk Reference*, the FDA website, CancerSource.com Drug Guide, and, in some cases, specific pharmaceutical companies' websites. Not all known side effects are listed here; consult with your doctor if you are experiencing side effects, whether they are listed here or not. Many of these medications also have interactions with other medications that produce symptoms not listed here.

Table 1 Drugs Used in the Treatment of Breast Cancer (continued)

Drug Name Generic (Brand), Maker	Actions/Common Side Effects[*]
Epirubicin (Ellence) Pfizer	Epirubicin (Ellence) was approved by the FDA in 1999 to treat early-stage breast cancer after breast surgery (lumpectomy or mastectomy) in patients whose cancer has spread to the lymph nodes. Epirubicin helps reduce the likelihood that breast cancer will return and improves a patient's chances of survival. Epirubicin is given intravenously (through the vein) in combination with two other chemotherapy drugs, cyclophosphamide and fluorouracil. Side effects may include nausea, vomiting, diarrhea, inflammation of the mouth, hair loss, damage to the skin if drug gets out of the veins, and reduction in white blood cells. Less common side effects: There is a risk of irreversible damage to the heart muscle associated with the drug. For women who receive epirubicin as adjuvant therapy, there is a slightly increased risk of treatment-related leukemia. Epirubicin may cause harm to the fetus if taken while pregnant.
ANTIMETA-BOLITES	**Antimetabolites prevent cells from making DNA and RNA by interfering with the synthesis of nucleic acids, thus disrupting the growth of cancer cells.**
5-Fluorouracil (5-FU, Adrucil, Fluorouracil) multiple makers	5-Fluorouracil is a drug that kills cancer cells by stopping their growth. It can also make it hard for cancer cells to fix damage. Side effects may include decreased white blood cell count with increased risk of infection; decreased platelet count with increased risk of bleeding; drowsiness or confusion; darkening of skin and nail beds; dry, flaky skin; nausea; vomiting; sores in mouth or on lips; thinning hair; diarrhea; brittle nails; and increased sensitivity to sun. Less common side effects: darkening and stiffening of vein used for giving the drug, decreased appetite, headache, weakness, and muscle aches. Cardiac symptoms are rare, but are most likely in patients with ischemic heart disease.
Capecitabine (Xeloda) Roche	Capecitabine (Xeloda) is approved as a treatment for advanced breast cancer. Capecitabine works by converting to 5-fluorouracil (5-FU) in the body. It is used for cancers resistant to both paclitaxel and anthracyclines. Side effects may include diarrhea, nausea, vomiting, loss of appetite or decreased appetite and dehydration, sores in mouth or on lips, numbness, tingling, itching of hands and/or feet, skin redness, rash, dryness, decreased white blood cell count with increased risk of infection, decreased platelet count with increased risk of bleeding, decreased red blood cell count with increased risk of fatigue, and irritation of the skin. Less common side effects: abdominal pain, constipation, heartburn after eating, fever, sensation of pins and needles in hands and/or feet, headache, dizziness, difficulty falling asleep, eye irritation, and increased value of blood tests for liver function.

[*]Drug information has been drawn from *The Physicians' Desk Reference*, the FDA website, CancerSource.com Drug Guide, and, in some cases, specific pharmaceutical companies' websites. Not all known side effects are listed here; consult with your doctor if you are experiencing side effects, whether they are listed here or not. Many of these medications also have interactions with other medications that produce symptoms not listed here.

Drug Name Generic (Brand), Maker	Actions/Common Side Effects*
Gemcitabine (Gemzar) Lilly Oncology	Gemcitabine (Gemzar) is approved as a treatment for advanced breast cancer in combination with paclitaxel. Side effects may include decreased blood counts with increased risk of infection, bleeding, and fatigue; nausea; vomiting; and skin rash. Less common side effects: fever, flu-like symptoms, swelling (edema), hair loss, and itching.
Ixabepilone (Ixempra) Bristol-Myers Squibb	Ixabepilone is approved for the treatment of aggressive monastic or locally advanced breast cancer no longer responding to currently available chemotherapies. Ixabepilone is administered through injection, in combination with capecitabine for the treatment of advanced breast cancer in patients after failure of an anthracycline and a taxane.
Methotrexate (MTX, Amethopterin, Folex, Mexate) multiple makers	Methotrexate prevents cells from making DNA and RNA by interfering with the synthesis of nucleic acids, thus stopping the growth of cancer cells. Side effects may include nausea (high dose), vomiting (high dose), sores in mouth or on lips, diarrhea, increased risk of sunburn, radiation recall skin changes, and loss of appetite. Less common side effects: decreased white blood cell count with increased risk of infection, decreased platelet count with increased risk of bleeding, and kidney damage (high dose). Liver, lung, and nerve damage are sometimes seen with methotrexate use, but the adjuvant drug, leucovorin, offsets the worst side effects.
MICROTUBULAR INHIBITOR	
Eribulin mesylate (Halaven) Eisai Inc	Halaven is a synthetic form of a chemotherapeutically active compound derived from the sea sponge *Halichondria okadai*. This injectable therapy is a microtubule inhibitor, believed to work by inhibiting cancer cell growth. Before receiving Halaven, patients should have received prior anthracycline- and taxane-based chemotherapy for early or late-stage breast cancer. It is an FDA-approved therapy used to treat late-stage aggressive breast cancer that is no longer responding to other chemotherapy agents. Halaven's safety and effectiveness were established in a single study in 762 women with metastatic breast cancer who had received at least two prior chemotherapy regimens for late-stage disease. Patients were randomly assigned to receive treatment with either Halaven or a different single agent therapy chosen by their oncologist. The study was designed to measure the length of time from when this treatment started until a patient's death (overall survival). The median overall survival for patients receiving Halaven was 13.1 months compared with 10.6 months for those who received a single agent therapy. The most common side effects reported by women treated with Halaven include a decrease in infection-fighting white blood cells (neutropenia), anemia, a decrease in the number of white blood cells (leukopenia), hair loss (alopecia), fatigue, nausea, weakness (asthenia), nerve damage (peripheral neuropathy), and constipation.

*Drug information has been drawn from *The Physicians' Desk Reference*, the FDA website, CancerSource.com Drug Guide, and, in some cases, specific pharmaceutical companies' websites. Not all known side effects are listed here; consult with your doctor if you are experiencing side effects, whether they are listed here or not. Many of these medications also have interactions with other medications that produce symptoms not listed here.

Table 1 Drugs Used in the Treatment of Breast Cancer (continued)

Drug Name Generic (Brand), Maker	Actions/Common Side Effects[*]
TAXANES	**Taxanes are powerful drugs that can stop cancer cells from repairing themselves and making new cells. Often used for treatment of cancers that have not responded to or have recurred after anthracycline therapy.**
Docetaxel (Taxotere) Sanofi-Aventis	The FDA has approved docetaxel to be used as a single agent over a wide range of doses, for the treatment of locally advanced or metastatic breast cancer in patients that have received prior chemotherapy. Docetaxel is also approved in combination with doxorubicin and cyclophosphamide for the adjuvant treatment of patients with operable, node-positive breast cancer. Docetaxel inhibits the division of breast cancer cells by acting on the cell's internal skeleton. Side effects may include decreased white blood cell count with increased risk of infection, decreased platelet count with increased risk of bleeding, hair thinning or loss, diarrhea, loss of appetite, nausea, vomiting, rash, and numbness and tingling in hands and/or feet related to peripheral nerve irritation or damage. Less common side effects: sores in mouth or on lips, swelling of ankles or hands, increased weight due to fluid retention, fatigue, muscle aches, loss of nails, and redness or irritation of the palms of hands or soles of feet.
Paclitaxel (Taxol) Bristol-Myers Squibb	Paclitaxel (Taxol) was first approved by the FDA in 1992 to treat advanced (metastatic) breast cancer. In 1999, the FDA also approved paclitaxel to treat early stage breast cancer in patients who have already received chemotherapy with the drug, doxorubicin. Paclitaxel is called a mitotic inhibitor because of its interference with cells during mitosis (cell division). Side effects may include decreased white blood cell count with increased risk of infection, fatigue, numbness and tingling in hands and/or feet related to peripheral nerve irritation or damage, muscle and bone aches for 3 days, hair loss, nausea, vomiting, mild diarrhea, and mild stomatitis. Less common side effects: allergic reaction: skin rash, flushing, increased heart rate, wheezing, and swelling of face. Transient heart problems such as bradycardia occur in 30 percent or less of patients and are usually not severe.
VINCA ALKALOIDS	**A medication in a class of anticancer drugs that inhibits cancer cell growth by stopping cell division (mitosis).**
Vinorelbine (Navelbine) GlaxoSmithKline	Vinorelbine (Navelbine) is used to treat metastatic breast cancer. Side effects may include decreased blood counts with increased risk of infection, and damage to the skin if drug gets outside the vein. Less common side effects: numbness and tingling of hands and feet, nausea, and vomiting.

[*]Drug information has been drawn from *The Physicians' Desk Reference*, the FDA website, CancerSource.com Drug Guide, and, in some cases, specific pharmaceutical companies' websites. Not all known side effects are listed here; consult with your doctor if you are experiencing side effects, whether they are listed here or not. Many of these medications also have interactions with other medications that produce symptoms not listed here.

Drug Name Generic (Brand), Maker	Actions/Common Side Effects[*]
TARGETED THERAPY	Targeted therapy is a general term that refers to a medication or drug that targets a specific pathway in the growth and development of a tumor. By attacking or blocking these important targets, the therapy helps to fight the tumor itself.
MONOCLONAL ANTIBODIES (BIOLOGIC AGENTS)	**Monoclonal antibodies work by attaching to a specific protein on cancer cells like a key in a lock, potentially creating an immune response that can help kill the cancer cells. Biologic agents are drugs produced from living organisms or cells. Some targeted therapies are biologics.**
Herceptin® (Trastuzumab) Genentech	Herceptin® (Trastuzumab) is an FDA-approved therapeutic for HER2 protein overexpressing metastatic breast cancer. Trastuzumab is a therapy for women with metastatic breast cancer whose tumors have too much HER2 protein. For patients with this disease, trastuzumab is approved for first-line use in combination with paclitaxel, and as a single agent for those who have received one or more chemotherapy regimens. Possible serious side effects include development of certain heart problems, including congestive heart failure; severe allergic reactions; infusion reactions; lung problems; blood clots; or a reduction in white blood cells. Side effects may include: fatigue, infections, low white or red blood cell counts, trouble breathing, rash/skin blistering, constipation, headache, and muscle pain.
Tykerb® (lapatinib)	Tykerb® (lapatinib) is used to treat advanced or metastatic breast cancer that overexpresses the HER2 protein. It is usually given in combination with capecitabine, after prior therapies. Possible serious side effects include development of lung problems and certain heart problems, including congestive heart failure. More common side effects may include rash, skin blistering, diarrhea, indigestion, nausea, vomiting, liver problems, anemia, bleeding or bruising, backache, arm or leg pain, problems sleeping, and shortness of breath.
ADJUVANT THERAPY	A variety of drugs that complement the chemotherapy regimen.
Leucovorin	Leucovorin is a form of vitamin used to offset the side effects of methotrexate and/or enhance the action of 5-FU. Leucovorin has few side effects itself, but its use with 5-FU can sometimes exacerbate the side effects of that drug.

[*]Drug information has been drawn from *The Physicians' Desk Reference*, the FDA website, CancerSource.com Drug Guide, and, in some cases, specific pharmaceutical companies' websites. Not all known side effects are listed here; consult with your doctor if you are experiencing side effects, whether they are listed here or not. Many of these medications also have interactions with other medications that produce symptoms not listed here.

Table 1 Drugs Used in the Treatment of Breast Cancer (continued)

Drug Name Generic (Brand), Maker	Actions/Common Side Effects*
Pamidronate (Aredia) Novartis Zoledronic acid (Zometa) Novartis Granisetron hydrochloride (Kytril) Dolasetron mesylate (Anzemet) Ondansetron hydro-chloride (Zofran) Palonosetron (Aloxi)	Both drugs are used to alleviate hypercalcemia; zoledronic acid is a newer, more powerful agent. Both drugs have similar side effects, which may include fever lasting for a short time (24–48 hours after infusion), pain at place of injection, and irritation of the vein used for giving the drug. Less common side effects: nausea, constipation, anemia, and decreased appetite. Renal function should be monitored with use of zoledronic acid. Zoledronic acid can cause bone damage (osteonecrosis) in the jaw.
Substance P/neuroki-nin (NK$_1$) receptor antagonist Aprepitant (Emend) Merck	Substance P/NK1 receptor antagonists block nausea and vomiting pathways. They are given with a serotonin antagonist and dexamethasone to prevent nausea and vomiting.

*Drug information has been drawn from *The Physicians' Desk Reference*, the FDA website, CancerSource.com Drug Guide, and, in some cases, specific pharmaceutical companies' websites. Not all known side effects are listed here; consult with your doctor if you are experiencing side effects, whether they are listed here or not. Many of these medications also have interactions with other medications that produce symptoms not listed here.

Table 2 Hormonal Therapies Used in Breast Cancer Treatment

Drug Name Generic (Brand), Maker	Type/Effects	Used For
Anastrozole (Arimidex®) AstraZeneca Pharmaceuticals	Aromatase inhibitor (reversible); prevents production of estrogen in adrenal glands	Initial treatment of postmenopausal women with hormone receptor-positive or hormone receptor-unknown locally advanced or metastatic breast cancer and for the treatment of postmenopausal women with advanced breast cancer that has progressed following treatment with tamoxifen.
Exemestane (Aromasin) Pfizer	Aromatase inhibitor (irreversible)	Adjuvant treatment of advanced breast cancer in postmenopausal women who have received 2–3 years of tamoxifen and are switched to exemestane to complete the 5 years of tamoxifen therapy.
Fulvestrant injection (Faslodex®) AstraZeneca Pharmaceuticals	Estrogen receptor antagonist	Treatment of hormone receptor-positive metastatic breast cancer in postmenopausal women with disease progression following anti-estrogen therapy. Research has confirmed that taking a higher dosage (500 mg) of this hormonal therapy than previously used may improve the clinical outcomes, slowing or stopping the progression of the disease.
Letrozole (Femara) Novartis Pharmaceuticals		Adjuvant treatment of postmenopausal women with hormone receptor positive early breast cancer. The effectiveness of Femara in early breast cancer is based on an analysis of disease-free survival in patients treated for a median of 24 months and followed for a median of 26 months. Follow up analyses will determine long-term outcomes for both safety and efficacy. Femara is also used for the extended adjuvant treatment of early breast cancer in postmenopausal women who have received 5 years of adjuvant tamoxifen therapy. The effectiveness of Femara in extended adjuvant treatment of early breast cancer is based on an analysis of disease-free survival in patients treated for a median of 24 months. Further data will be required to determine long-term outcome. Femara is also used for first-line treatment of postmenopausal women with hormone receptor positive or hormone receptor unknown locally advanced or metastatic breast cancer.

(continues)

Table 2 Hormonal Therapies Used in Breast Cancer Treatment (continued)

Drug Name Generic (Brand), Maker	Type/Effects	Used For
Letrozole (Femara) Novartis Pharmaceuticals (continued)	Aromatase inhibitor (reversible)	Femara is also indicated for the treatment of advanced breast cancer in postmenopausal women with disease progression following anti-estrogen therapy.
Megestrol acetate (Megace) Bristol-Myers Squibb	Aromatase inhibitor; mimics action of progesterone, blocking it from progesterone receptors	Used to treat PR+ cancers. Because it is also an appetite stimulant, may be preferred for underweight patients who have responsive cancers.
Tamoxifen citrate	Binds to estrogen receptors, blocking estrogen from the cancer cells	Tamoxifen citrate is effective in the treatment of metastatic breast cancer in women and men. In premenopausal women with metastatic breast cancer, tamoxifen citrate is an alternative to oophorectomy or ovarian irradiation. Available evidence indicated that patients whose tumors are estrogen receptor positive are more likely to benefit from tamoxifen citrate therapy. **Adjuvant Treatment of Breast Cancer:** tamoxifen citrate is indicated for the treatment of node-positive breast cancer in postmenopausal women following total mastectomy or segmental mastectomy, axillary dissection, and breast irradiation. Tamoxifen citrate is also indicated for the treatment of axillary node-negative breast cancer in women following total mastectomy or segmental mastectomy, axillary dissection, and breast irradiation. In addition, tamoxifen citrate reduces the occurrence of contralateral breast cancer in patients receiving adjuvant therapy with tamoxifen citrate for breast cancer. **Ductal Carcinoma in Situ (DCIS):** In women with DCIS, following breast surgery and radiation, tamoxifen citrate is indicated to reduce the risk of invasive breast cancer. (See **BOXED WARNING** at the beginning of full Prescribing Information.) *(continues)*

Drug Name Generic (Brand), Maker	Type/Effects	Used For
Tamoxifen citrate (continued)	Binds to estrogen receptors, blocking estrogen from the cancer cells	**Reduction in Breast Cancer Incidence in High Risk Women:** tamoxifen citrate is indicated to reduce the incidence of breast cancer in women at high risk for breast cancer. Tamoxifen citrate is indicated only for high-risk women. "High risk" is defined as women at least 35 years of age with a 5-year predicted risk of breast cancer ≥ 1.67%, as calculated by the Gail Model. (See **BOXED WARNING** at the beginning of full Prescribing Information.)
Toremifene citrate (Fareston) Orion Corporation	Aromatase inhibitor	Treatment of metastatic breast cancer in postmenopausal women with ER+ or receptor-unknown tumors.

Resources to Benefit Breast Cancer Patients and Their Families

American Cancer Society
(800) ACS-2345
www.cancer.org/docroot/home/
    index.asp

America's Health Insurance Plans
601 Pennsylvania Ave NW,
    South Bldg, Suite 500
Washington, DC 20004
(202) 778-3200
ahip@ahip.org
www.ahip.org

ASCO—American Society of Clinical Oncology
American Society of Clinical
    Oncology
1900 Duke Street, Suite 200
Alexandria, VA 22314
(703) 299-0150
asco@asco.org
www.asco.org

Breastcancer.org
(610) 642-6550
comments@breastcancer.org
www.breastcancer.org

Breast Cancer Network of Strength
(800) 221-2141
    (24-hour national hotline)
(800) 986-9505
    (24-hour hotline in Spanish)
Email: info@y-me.org
www.networkofstrength.org

Cancer Care, Inc.
(800) 813-HOPE
info@cancercare.org
www.cancercare.org

Cancer Research Institute
(800) 99-CANCER
www.cancerresearch.org

CenterWatch Clinical Trials Listing Service
22 Thomson Place, 47F1
Boston, MA 02210-1212
(617) 856-5900
www.centerwatch.com/patient/
    trials.html

**Financial Planning
Association**
1600 K Street NW
Washington, DC 20006
(800) 282-75296
www.fpanet.org

**The Johns Hopkins Avon
Foundation Breast Center**
www.hopkinsbreastcenter.org

Living Beyond Breast Cancer
354 W. Lancaster Ave, Suite 224
Haverford, PA 19041
National Helpline
(888) 753-5222
(484) 708-1550
mail@lbbc.org
www.lbbc.org

**Metastatic Breast Cancer
Network**
(888) 500-0370
mbcnet@gmail.com

**Mothers Supporting
Daughters with Breast Cancer
(MSDBC)**
(410) 778-1982
msdbc@verizon.net
www.mothersdaughters.org

**National Breast Cancer
Coalition**
1101 17th Street, NW,
Suite 1300
Washington, DC 20036
(800) 622-2838
(202) 265-6854
www.StopBreastCancer.org

National Cancer Institute
Public Office of Information
Building 31, Room 10A31
31 Center Drive, MSC 2580
Bethesda, MD 20892-2580
(800) 4-CANCER
www.cancer.gov

**National Center for
Complementary and
Alternative Medicine**
(888) 644-6226
info@nccam.nih.gov
www.nccam.nih.gov

**National Comprehensive
Cancer Network**
(888) 909-NCCN
www.nccn.org

National Institutes of Health
National Institutes of Health
9000 Rockville Pike
Bethesda, Maryland 20892
(301) 496-4000
NIHInfo@do.nih.gov
www.nih.gov
www.clinicaltrials.gov (for information on clinical trials)

National Consortium of Breast Centers
PO Box 1334
Warsaw, IN 46581-1334
(574) 267-8058
ncbc@breastcare.org
www.breastcare.org/ or
    www.ncbcinc.org/

National Lymphedema Network
Latham Square
1611 Telegraph Ave, Suite 111
Oakland, CA 94612-2138
(800) 541-3259
    or (510) 208-3200
NLN@lymphnet.org
www.lymphnet.org

Society of Surgical Oncology
www.surgonc.org

Susan G. Komen for the Cure
National Helpline
    (800) IM-AWARE
www.breastcancerinfo.com

Young Survival Coalition
61 Broadway, Suite 2235
New York, NY 10006
(877) YSC-1011
(646) 257-3000
info@youngsurvival.org
www.youngsurvival.org

Where can I get help with financial or legal concerns?

Accompanying any serious illness are questions and concerns related to expenses incurred as a result of treatment, health insurance questions that can be overwhelming to try to understand or resolve alone, and sometimes even legal questions related to employment or financial matters. This list of national resources can aid you in addressing your concerns.

America's Health Insurance Plans
601 Pennsylvania Ave NW,
    South Bldg, Suite 500
Washington, DC 20004
(202) 778-3200
ahip@ahip.org
www.ahip.org

Cancer Care, Inc.
(800) 813-HOPE
info@cancercare.org
www.cancercare.org

Credit Counseling Centers of America/ Money Management International
(800) 493-2222
www.cccamerica.org

Hill-Burton Free Care Program
(800) 638-0742
In MD, call (800) 492-0359
www.hrsa.gov/hillburton/
    compliance-recovery.htm

National Association of Hospital Hospitality Houses, Inc.
PO Box 18087
Asheville, NC 22814-0087
(800) 542-9730
(828) 253-1188
helpinghomes@nahhh.org
www.nahhh.org

National Coalition for Cancer Survivorship (NCCS)
1010 Wayne Ave, Suite 770
Silver Spring, MD 20910
(888) 650-9127
(301) 650-9127
info@ccansearch.org
www.canceradvocacy.org

Patient Advocate Foundation
700 Thimble Shoals Blvd,
    Suite 200
Newport News, VA 23606
(800) 532-5274
(757) 873-6668
help@patientadvocate.org
www.patientadvocate.org

Social Security Administration
Office of Public Inquiries
(800) 772-1213
www.ssa.gov

A

Acupuncture: The technique of inserting thin needles into the skin at specific points. This can help control pain and other symptoms for some individuals and is a form of ancient Chinese medicine. It is a form of complementary therapy.

Adjuncts: Drugs that complement the chemotherapy regimen.

Adjuvant therapy: Treatment given after the primary treatment to increase the chances of a cure, and treatment to prevent the cancer from recurring.

Adjuvant studies: A clinical trial to determine if additional therapy will further opportunity for survival.

Advanced directives: Legal documents that allow people to express their decisions regarding what they do and don't want to have done during their last weeks or months in case they become unable to communicate effectively.

Alternative medicine: Medicines used in lieu of standard medical therapies.

Analgesic: Drugs that reduce pain.

Anemia: A condition in which the number of red blood cells is too low.

Antibodies: Special proteins produced by your immune system. They help protect the body from disease.

Antigens: Specific cells that substances that are not supposed to be in your body (like viruses, bacteria, or cell changes that are very abnormal) produce.

Antiemetics: Drugs to stop or prevent nausea or vomiting.

Aromatase inhibitor: Drugs that lower the amount of estrogen made in the body after menopause. This can slow or stop the growth of cancer that needs estrogen to grow.

Ascites: A buildup of fluid in the abdominal cavity.

Asymptomatic: Not manifesting any symptoms.

Axillary lymph node dissection: Removal of lymph nodes in the armpit during the initial surgery; the nodes are then examined by a pathologist to determine if cancerous cells are present.

B

Biopsy: A procedure in which cells are collected for microscopic examination.

Blood-brain barrier: A special layer that protects the brain from infection. This layer is made up of a network of blood vessels with thick walls.

Bone density (DEXA) scan: A test to evaluate bone mineral density. The results predict the likelihood of fracture. The DEXA scan calculates bone density based on the amount of radiation absorbed by the bone, and compares your bone strength with that of young premenopausal women.

Bone scan: An X-ray that looks for signs of metastasis to the bones.

Breast cancer case conference: Same as tumor board. A special meeting of oncology doctors and nurses for the purpose of discussing a specific patient's case and planning a recommended treatment. Usually involves the review of pathology slides, mammograms, other X-rays, and a discussion about what would be the best course of action for treating the patient's breast cancer.

Breast cancer tumor board: Same as case conference. A special meeting of oncology doctors and nurses for the purpose of discussing a specific patient's case and planning a recommended treatment. Usually involves the review of pathology slides, mammograms, other X-rays, and a discussion about what would be the best course of action for treating the patient's breast cancer.

Breast mass: An abnormal collection of tissue within the breast.

C

Complementary and alternative medicine (CAM): Forms of treatment that are used in addition to, or instead of, standard treatments. Their purpose is to strengthen your whole mind and body to maximize your health, energy, and well-being. These practices are not considered "standard" medical approaches. They include dietary supplements, vitamins, herbal preparations, special teas, massage therapy, acupuncture, spiritual healing, visualization, and meditation.

Cancer: The presence of malignant cells.

Cells: Basic elements of tissues; the appearance and composition of individual cells are unique to the tissue they compose.

Chemotherapy: Treatment with drugs that kill cancer cells or make them less active. It is a form of systemic treatment.

Clinical trials: Research studies in which patients are offered the opportunity to try new innovative therapies (under careful observation) in order to help doctors identify the best treatments with the fewest side effects. These studies help improve the overall standard of care.

Combination chemotherapy: Treatment using more than one anti-cancer drug at a time.

Complementary therapy: Medicines used in conjunction with standard therapies.

Cytotoxic: A term used to describe anything that kills cells.

D

Distant recurrence: The breast cancer has been found now in another organ, such as the lungs, liver, bones, or brain. It is located outside of the breast and lymph nodes near the breast.

E

ECHO test: A special test using ultrasound that determines the strength of the heart.

EGFR (epidermal growth factor receptor): The receptor protein found on the surface of some cells and to which the epidermal growth factor binds, causing the cells to divide. EGFR appears to be a cancer stimulant, found at abnormally high levels on the surface of many types of cancer cells, and may be why these cells divide excessively if the epidermal growth factor is also present.

Estrogen: Female hormone related to child bearing.

Estrogen-receptor positive cancer: A cancer that grows more rapidly with exposure to the hormone estrogen.

F

First-line therapy: The first drug or set of drugs that you receive as your treatment.

FISH (Fluorescence in situ hybridization): This is a lab test that measures the amount of a certain gene in cells. It can be used to see if an invasive cancer has too many HER2 genes. A cancer with too many of these genes is called HER2-positive.

G

Growth factor receptor: The receptor protein found on the surface of some cells and to which the epidermal growth factor binds, causing the cells to divide. EGFR appears to be a cancer stimulant, found at abnormally high levels on the surface of many types of cancer cells, and may be why these cells divide excessively if the epidermal growth factor is also present.

Guided imagery: A mind body technique in which the patient visualizes and meditates upon images that encourage a positive immune response.

H

Healthcare proxy: Permits a designated person to make decisions regarding your medical treatment when you are unable to do so.

Hemoglobin: The part of the red blood cell that carries the oxygen.

HER2 overexpression: An excess of a certain protein (HER2) on the surface of a cell that may be related to a high number of abnormal or defective cells.

Hormonal therapy: Treatment that blocks the effects of hormones upon cancers that depend on hormones to grow (also referred to as endocrine therapy).

Hormone receptors: A protein on the surface or inside a cell that connects to a certain hormone (estrogen or progesterone) and causes changes in the cell.

Hormone replacement therapy: Administration of artificial estrogen and progesterone to alleviate the symptoms of menopause and to prevent health problems experienced by postmenopausal women, particularly osteoporosis.

Hospice: An organization that provides programs and services designed to help alleviate the physical and psychosocial suffering associated with progressive, incurable illness.

Hypercalcemia: Accelerated loss of calcium in bones, leading to elevated levels of the mineral in the bloodstream with symptoms such as nausea and confusion.

I

Immunohistochemistry (IHC): The most commonly used test to see if a tumor has too much of the HER2 receptor protein on the surface of the cancer cells. The IHC test gives a score of 0 to 3+ that indicates the amount of HER2 receptor protein. It also measures the presence of hormone receptors on the breast cancer cell too and determines if a tumor is hormone receptor positive or negative.

Incidence: The number of times a disease occurs within a population of people.

K

Ki67: A molecule that can be easily detected in growing cells in order to gain an understanding of the rate at which the cells within a tumor are growing.

L

Living will: Outlines what care you want in the event you become unable to communicate due to coma or heavy sedation.

Locally advanced disease: Stage III breast cancer. Cancer that is in a large area of the breast and lymph nodes under the arm; it may be fixed on the chest wall.

Local recurrence: The breast cancer has returned inside the breast after treatment was completed.

Local treatment: Refers to anything that is targeted to a specific area of the body—such as the breast, the lymph nodes, the lungs—as opposed to the whole body.

Lumpectomy: Breast cancer surgery to remove the breast cancer and a small amount of normal tissue surrounding it.

Lymph: Fluid carried through the body by the lymphatic system, composed primarily of white blood cells and diluted plasma.

Lymph nodes: Tissues in the lymphatic system that filter lymph fluid and help the immune system fight disease.

Lymphatic system: A collection of vessels with the principal functions of transporting digested fat from the intestine to the bloodstream, removing and destroying toxins from tissues, and resisting the spread of disease throughout the body.

Lymphedema: A condition in which lymph fluid collects in tissues following removal of, or damage to, lymph nodes during surgery, causing the limb or area of the body affected to swell.

M

Malignant: Cancerous; growing rapidly and out of control.

Mammogram: An X-ray examination of the breast.

Mastectomy: Surgery that removes the whole breast.

Medical oncologist: See oncologist.

Meditation: A mental technique that clears the mind and relaxes the body through concentration.

Menopause: End of menstrual periods.

Metastases, metastasize: The spread of cancer from one part of the body to another.

Metastatic breast cancer: Cancer that has spread from the breast to other organ sites such as the liver, lung, bone, or brain.

Micrometastases: Small numbers of cancer cells that have spread from the primary tumor to other parts of the body and are too few to be picked up in a screening or diagnostic test.

Mucositis: A condition in which the mucosa (the lining of the digestive tract, from the mouth to the anus) becomes swollen, red, and sore. For example, sores in the mouth that can be a side effect of chemotherapy.

MUGA test: A special test that determines the strength of the heart and is given for women having chemotherapy or targeted therapy that may cause heart problems as a complication.

N

Nadir: The low point of blood counts that occurs as a result of chemotherapy.

Neutropenia: An abnormally low number of a particular type of white blood cell called a neutrophil. White blood cells (leukocytes) are the cells in the blood that play important roles by fighting off infection.

Neutropenic fever: A fever due to a low white blood cell count, usually caused by a side effect of chemotherapy.

Noninvasive cancer: Cancer confined to its tissue point of origin and not found in surrounding tissues.

Nonsteroidal anti-inflammatory drugs (NSAIDs): A class of pain medications, often sold over-the-counter, that includes ibuprofen and similar common pain killers.

O

Oncologist: A cancer specialist who helps determine treatment choices.

Osteonecrosis: When some non-cancerous bone cells die off in a way that is not normal.

Osteopenia: A condition of less bone density or bone mass than would be normally expected if you compare a woman to a woman or population of women her age. It is the bone loss that, if it continues, can lead to osteoporosis.

Overall survival: The percentage of people in a study who have survived for a certain period of time, usually reported as time since diagnosis or treatment. Often called the survival rate.

P

Palliative care: Care to relieve the symptoms of cancer and to keep the best quality of life for as long as possible without seeking to cure cancer.

Paracentesis: A procedure to take out fluid that has collected in the abdominal cavity. This fluid buildup, called ascites, may be caused by infection, inflammation, an injury, or other conditions, such as cancer. The fluid is taken out using a long, thin needle put through the belly. The fluid is sent to a lab and studied to find the cause of the fluid buildup. Paracentesis also may be done to take the fluid out to relieve belly pressure or pain in people with cancer or cirrhosis.

Pathologist: A specialist trained to distinguish normal from abnormal cells.

Patient Navigators: An individual who assists patients in navigating their care and treatment by assisting them with scheduling appointments, answering questions related to test results, patient education, support, and providing guidance in decision-making across the continuum of care.

Peripheral neuropathy: Numbness and pain of the hands and feet, which can be caused by infection, very strong drugs (such as chemotherapy), or disease.

Phases: A series of steps followed in clinical trials.

Placebos: A pill or treatment that looks the same and is taken in the same way as a drug or treatment in a clinical trial, but contains no active drug ingredients.

Plastic surgeon: A surgical specialist who will perform any reconstruction procedures that might be required.

Platelets: Components of blood that assist in clotting and wound healing.

Pleurodesis: A procedure that gets rid of the open space between the lung and the chest cavity. This is done to stop fluid from building up in this space. When cancer cells are growing in this space, they make fluid that can collect and cause difficulty breathing. During this surgery, a chemical is placed in the space. Your body's reaction to the chemical causes the lining around the lung to stick to the inside lining of the chest wall.

Pleural cavity: A space between the outside of the lungs and the inside wall of the chest cavity.

Port: The treatment site.

Primary care doctor: A regular physician who gives checkups.

Progesterone-receptor positive cancer: Cancer that grows more rapidly with exposure to the hormone progesterone.

Progestin: A synthetic form of progesterone often used in birth control pills and hormone replacement therapy.

Prognosis: An estimation of the likely outcome of an illness based upon the patient's current status and the available treatments.

Progression-free survival: The length of time during and after treatment in which a patient is living with a disease that does not get worse. Progression-free survival may be used in a clinical study or trial to help find out how well a new treatment works

Protocols: The research plan for how the drug is given and to whom it is given.

R

Radiologist: A physician who specializes in radiology which includes reading of X-rays, scans, and other imaging studies used to diagnose various conditions and diseases.

Radiation oncologist: A cancer specialist who determines the amount of radiotherapy required.

Radiation physicist: Makes sure that the equipment is working properly and that the machines deliver the right dose of radiation.

Radiation therapy: The use of high-energy X-rays to kill cancer cells and shrink tumors.

Randomized: Describes the process in a clinical trial in which animal or human subjects are assigned by chance to separate groups that allow for comparison of different treatments.

Recurrent cancer: The disease has come back in spite of the initial treatment.

Red blood cells (RBCs): Cells in the blood with the primary function of carrying oxygen to tissues.

Remission: A decrease in or disappearance of signs and symptoms of cancer. In partial remission, some, but not all, signs and symptoms have disappeared. In complete remission, all signs and symptoms have disappeared, although there may still be cancer cells present in the body.

Risk factors: Any factors that contribute to an increased possibility of getting cancer.

S

Scans: A technique to create images of specific parts of the body on a computer screen or on film.

Stage: A numerical determination of how far the cancer has progressed.

Standard of care: A diagnostic and treatment process that a clinician should follow for a certain type of patient, illness, or clinical circumstances.

Surgical oncologist: A specialist trained in surgical removal of cancerous tumors.

Systemic treatment: A treatment that affects the whole body (the patient's whole system).

T

Targeted therapy: Treatments for breast cancer that target specific characteristics of cancer cells, such as a protein, an enzyme, or the formation of new blood cells. Targeted therapies don't harm normal, healthy cells. Most are antibodies that work like the antibodies made by the immune system. They are not chemotherapy.

Thoracentesis: The removal of fluid from the pleural cavity through a hollow needle inserted between the ribs.

Total (simple) mastectomy: When a surgeon removes the whole breast but does not remove lymph nodes.

Transverse rectus abdominus muscle (TRAM) flap: A muscle from the abdomen, along with skin and fat, is transferred to the mastectomy site and shaped like a breast, see also breast reconstruction.

Tumor: A mass or lump of extra tissue.

U

Ultrasound: Uses sound waves to determine whether a lump is solid or filled with fluid.

Uterine cancer: A cancer beginning in the uterus; sometimes related genetically to breast cancer.

V

Vascular access device (VAD): A special catheter is inserted inside a major vein (generally in one of the large veins in the neck) extending into the large central vein near the heart so that blood can be repeatedly drawn or medication and nutrients can be injected into the patient's bloodstream on a continual basis or dialysis can be performed.

Vascular endothelial growth factor (VEGF): A substance made by cells that causes new blood vessels to form.